Eternal
Spring

of related interest

You Are How You Move
Experiential Chi Kung
Ged Sumner
978 1 84819 014 6

Tàijí Jiàn 32-Posture Sword Form
James Drewe
ISBN 978 1 84819 011 5

Meet Your Body
A Rolfer's Guide to Releasing Bodymindcore Trauma
Noah Karrasch
ISBN 978 1 84819 016 0

TAIJIQUAN, QI GONG, AND THE CULTIVATION
OF HEALTH, HAPPINESS AND LONGEVITY

Eternal Spring

Michael W. Acton

SINGING DRAGON
London and Philadelphia

First published in 2009
by Singing Dragon
An imprint of Jessica Kingsley Publishers
116 Pentonville Road
London N1 9JB, UK
and
400 Market Street, Suite 400
Philadelphia, PA 19106, USA

www.singing-dragon.com

Library of Congress Cataloging in Publication Data
Acton, Michael W., 1937-
Eternal spring : Taiji quan, Qi gong, and the cultivation of health, happiness, and longevity / Michael W. Acton.
p. cm.
ISBN 978-1-84819-003-0 (pb : alk. paper) 1. Happiness. 2. Longevity. 3. Health. 4. Tai chi. 5. Qi gong. I. Title.
BF575.H27.A28 2009
158'.90951–dc22

2008042442

British Library Cataloguing in Publication Data
A CIP catalogue record for this book is available from the British Library

ISBN 978 1 84819 003 0

Printed and bound in the United States by
Thomson-Shore, 7300 Joy Road, Dexter, MI 48130

Acknowledgements

To my guide and Master Dr Li Li Qun of Shanghai, who has set me on the clear path, and to my wife Suzie (Shao Qing) and my daughter India (Yue Ru) who have kindly put up with me. To my most dedicated students who have encouraged me to find the words, and finally to all who wish to gently push open the window and let in the light.

Contents

Preface

This book is the result of 30 years of practice, many of which were fruitless, and 16 years of study with a true master, Dr Li Li Qun of Shanghai (every moment of which has been a treasure). Master Li is a highly regarded fourth generation master of Wu Style Taiji boxing, a doctor of Traditional Chinese Medicine and a master of Qi Gong. He started studying Chinese boxing at the age of six and has studied many styles. Now in his eighties, he is both a bridge to the founding fathers of Taijiquan and an authority on the traditional styles, methods and meaning that are the ancient treasure of Chinese boxing and Qi Gong. I am privileged to be his 'disciple'.

This book can only express a small part of what I have learned but I hope it offers some insight into these precious arts, as well as conveying my firm belief, along with most of China, that the practice of Qi Gong and Taijiquan brings such significant benefits to health, happiness and ageing that it should become a major part of our health culture. Taught in schools it would provide a mental and physical discipline. Taught to the older generation it can rejuvenate and revitalise. Taught to the sick, it can offer relief and possible recovery as well as (and perhaps most important) active and positive participation in taking control of their own mental and physical well-being.

The practice of Qi Gong and Taijiquan is also self-empowering, since it not only brings physical health and mental well-being, but also engenders the courage to accept and understand our condition and the ebb and flow of our lives and to take responsibility for our own nature and actions. Its traditional strategies and methods are a blueprint for surviving the stresses and strains of our modern-day lives. The way of Qi Gong and Taijiquan is a path of self-discovery, achievement and fulfilment; it is the panacea for our time.

This book is not really instructional and neither is it an academic treatise. It is simply based upon my teaching experience and my own study and practice at the feet of a recognised master. Its aim is modest but I hope it can convey the essential principles, methods and meaning of these traditional arts. The promise of Taijiquan and Qi Gong is the promise of physical and mental health as well as Spiritual development. It is about 'nourishing life' by cultivating the mind, the body and the Spirit. It is about restoring, rejuvenating and maintaining your physical and mental health and vitality as long as you can. In China, this achievement is referred to colloquially as Eternal Spring.

Qi Gong and Taijiquan are an investment and a treasure for life.

I hope the following chapters serve as both an inspiration and an explanation of the fundamentals of these 'arts', for such they are. Like all good art they are a living expression of our life force, our knowledge, understanding and curiosity, and as true art they lead us to a deeper and more profound understanding of our condition and place in the world and beyond.

I have left out much that I would like to say but I have tried to keep what is a complex, wide and incredibly deep subject as simple and coherent as possible. You cannot travel this path by reading alone. You must undertake the physical and mental practice, but it helps to have some inspiration and guidance on how you should be thinking, what you should be studying, and why. I hope that this little book will suffice, at least until you are well on the way and have replaced my thoughts with your own experience.

Michael Acton (Li Shui)
London, June 2008

The World We Live In

The way we are

Our modern world is now a fast and fearsome place. We are inundated with systems and authorities, plagued by rules and bureaucracy, touted for memberships and exclusivities, offers and deals, and weighed down by the cost of living, property and education – or, for many, simply poverty. At work we must have an eye on our job security, be productive and seek opportunities, deal with redundancy, re-education, downsizing, and possibly retrain for a second career, or just struggle on and wonder what our old age will be like. It can often feel like a treadmill or a hopeless cause.

We all struggle to juggle our needs, the pressures and demands on us. We try to maintain an equilibrium but it takes very little to destabilise us and to expose the fragility of our health and emotional well-being. We tend to hurtle from one need to the next, firefighting on the way. We are driven by ambition, attraction, repulsion and a complex cocktail of habitual emotional and physical needs. We become increasingly anaesthetised to our mental and physical health, until what we take for granted, our minds and bodies, rebel under the strain. When we meet with crisis, poor health, mental overload or even death, we often realise how ill prepared we are to face life and just how much effort we have expended on everything else but ourselves, our health and our well-being.

We often long for a deeper and more meaningful connection with ourselves, others and our environment, but we are unable to extricate ourselves from the complex ties and forces that bind us to a particular course in life. We may search for a meaningful way of managing ourselves within our own context. We may try to find a job, change jobs, change career, find religion or often simply make small adjustments to our lives to help us cope and feel better. We may go on a diet, join a gym for the quick hit of 45 minutes twice a week, swim or play a game of golf or squash on Sundays, learn Yoga, Pilates or any of the myriad methods that have emerged in the gym and faddish healthy culture. These can all help, and many people rely on them to manage stress and to maintain fitness, as well as to look good in our fashion-conscious and anti-ageist society. But much of what is available now, although excellent, is often expensive, temporary and without deeper intellectual, physical or 'Spiritual' value. It is true that many people do not want to have to think about their health, lifestyle or workout, and believe the body can be maintained rather like a car and the mind kept happy by work and pleasure. Cars, however, can be replaced, whereas bodies and minds, at least for the moment, cannot.

There is now plenty of evidence that mental activity plays a critical role in our overall sense of physical and mental well-being. Certain types of exercise, for instance, when accompanied by appropriate mental activity, can have significant impact on the immune, lymphatic and nervous systems, as well as on the heart and blood pressure. Obesity, heart disease and other lifestyle-related illnesses, as well as anxiety-related disorders, are now prevalent in Western urban society, putting increasing pressure on limited resources. A free and achievable discipline like Qi Gong taught across whole populations could help to relieve that pressure. The ultimate exercise should engage all of us and infuse our whole life with a tangible quality of physical well-being, emotional equilibrium and mental clarity. It should both keep us healthy and enhance our 'inner' life. It should de-stress not just the daily tensions but the deeper, residual, cumulative tensions resulting from childhood, adolescence and becoming a fully formed individual in a complex and stressful adult world. It should act as a first defence against the onset of currently prevalent illness and disease, and strengthen both our resistance and resolve by helping us significantly adjust the factors that cause such illness.

Finally, it should be an investment for our old age. We would all like to grow old gracefully, retain as best we can our balance and co-ordination, our good health and vigour, our intellect and our independence. In China this is often referred to as 'Eternal Spring' and it is to the ancient culture of China and to a traditional Daoist martial art called Taijiquan and an ancient Daoist health and Spiritual practice called Qi Gong that we must turn. Created long ago and developed over centuries, these two disciplines have remarkable applicability to our modern condition. It is within these two disciplines that we find the means and knowledge necessary to truly enhance our lives and perhaps even lengthen them.

A bit of background

It was back in the early 1970s that I became fascinated with a little-known, and at that time little-understood form of Chinese boxing called Taijiquan. Associated mostly with old Chinese people dressed in workmen's blues, waving their arms around in slow motion, Taijiquan seemed to be both mundane and mysterious. It was variously called 'shadow boxing' and 'meditation in movement' and seemed to be found only amongst Chinese communities. Beyond the early Western pioneers of the oriental arts, most 'Westerners' who knew about or taught Taijiquan practised it as a sort of 'meditational dance', often devoid of any clear meaning or purpose. Those who taught its martial and health components often seemed unable to give Taijiquan a sense of authenticity or consensus of purpose, or even martial credibility. Taijiquan seemed to hang somewhere between a depleted martial art and an expression of Chinese health culture.

Taijiquan's close and historically older, but at that time little-known relative Qi Gong offered the secrets of extraordinary martial power as well as health, happiness and longevity. Qi Gong was slow to emerge as a serious health system and greater awareness did not take root properly outside the overseas Chinese communities until Chinese medicine became more widely adopted as a serious alternative for effective health care. The softer side of Qi Gong came to be recognised as a branch of Chinese medicine and, to the lucky few, a traditional Daoist means of Spiritual cultivation.

Both Taijiquan and Qi Gong share traditional and obscure Daoist roots. Both disciplines were commonly linked to a seminal Daoist work known as the *Dao De Jing*, written by Lao Tze (trans. Lau 1963). Though Daoist ideas and practice existed long before Lao Tze wrote his text, this document became the Western face of Daoism. It outlined a philosophy based on harmonising extremes, ambiguities and paradox; behaving naturally in accordance with prevailing conditions and cultivating a meditational mindset and balanced understanding of the ebb and flow of events, all of which should be understood or intuited as part of a bigger process. It offered advice to both rulers and individuals alike on virtuous behaviour and self-cultivation. It spoke of living in harmony, according to the rules of the 'Dao', the immutable laws of change, and it alluded to secret teachings for Spiritual cultivation. Needless to say, the cryptic nature of the text was open to serious misinterpretation, and indeed humour. It was often conjured by teachers to add value and mystery to the Taiji 'dance'.

In the mid 1970s the residue of the sixties still lingered. Transcendental Meditation (TM) had long gained respectability. A variety of therapies, Spiritual development, meditation and Yoga of various shades had blossomed. Japanese martial arts were dominant and their association with Zen was well understood. Indeed Zen was the new existentialism, and most self-respecting Spiritual intellectuals had read *Zen in the Art of Archery* by Eugen Herrigel (1989) and had the writings of D.T. Suzuki and Alan Watts on the shelf (see, for example, Suzuki 1961, 1964 and Watts 1997, 1999). The spiritual journey still generally started in Delhi and for the fighter, it started at the Budokwi (training room for Judo and Aikido) with its special mats and ritualised hierarchy and respectful bowing. Aikido's effortless style, beauty, humility and talk of Ki (Qi) was deeply mysterious. Karate was the choice of most young bloods and, with its promise of Katas (a set of martial movements practised solo for martial training), uniform and gradings, provided proof of ability. Karate and Judo were also popular competitive sports.

Regarding things Chinese, in the 1970s access to mainland China was still largely restricted to visitors from the outside world and so most knowledge in the West resided in America where, historically, many Chinese had migrated. The memorable portrayal of a Shaolin monk in the American television series called *Kung Fu* gave rise to an awareness of Spiritual, Zen-like dimensions in Chinese boxing, previously unknown. It framed the link between Zen and its mother, Chan Buddhism in China, and confirmed that those graceful, animal-related movements of Shaolin boxing were a previously hidden union of Chinese martial and religious culture.

Bruce Lee's film *Enter the Dragon* provided the muscle that brought Chinese boxing to the streets and the big screen and, though he talked in Spiritually charged aphorisms, the meaning of it all got lost in the ambition to Wing-Chun your way to martial superiority in your neighbourhood. Somehow the link between Zen and Japanese martial arts (especially Aikido) as a Spiritual, highly refined method of self-cultivation (as well as a way of cracking heads) was not reflected in the Chinese martial arts as exemplified by Bruce Lee. The power and muscle, speed and skill left the softer and esoteric side of inner cultivation back in the temple. It did not seem to come out for some time, and consequently the tradition of self-cultivation through refining the physical and mental self, that grew to such sophistication in China amongst Daoist and Buddhist adepts, and which greatly influenced the evolution of the martial arts, had no broad exposure and few mainstream proponents in the West at that time, outside the Chinese communities in America.

Nevertheless Bruce Lee and the Hong Kong cinema gave Chinese boxing (commonly called Kung Fu in the West) a new and high profile. Bruce Lee's own system, Jeet Kun Do, and one of its main roots, Wing Chun, took off commercially on the back of the exotic martial arts surge. Taijiquan, however, had few heroes then.

Now there is a plethora of Chinese martial arts teachers, teaching mainstream and previously obscure Chinese systems. There are now many teachers of Taijiquan and Qi Gong and indeed, like myself, some have lived and trained in China, Taiwan and Hong Kong with authentic masters. Consequently Taijiquan is now recognised as both a boxing art and a health practice, and Qi Gong has gained ground as a profound health and Spiritual practice.

This is good news, because for too long these Chinese disciplines have been viewed suspiciously by martial artists, health therapists and medical practitioners alike.

Taiji, however, is still publicly perceived as somehow lacking, since it suffers a dual personality. It is, on the one hand, a very refined martial art and on the other a sophisticated expression of Chinese health culture (Qi Gong) underpinned by Daoist natural philosophy. From the martial perspective, it is not embraced by military training, neither does it feature as an international or Olympic competitive sport (yet), nor is it a ring sport like Western boxing, and it is not seen in the Hong Hong 'Kung Fu' film genre. As a health modality it has not really entered the Western gym or medical culture in the way that Yoga and Pilates have. It is not, at least not yet, 'sexy' in an advertising sort of way, neither has it entered the public awareness as a significant method for personal fitness and mental well-being.

As disciplines, Taiji and Qi Gong also appear difficult to learn and to understand, which puts off large numbers who just wish to dip into a keep-fit regimen or learn a bit of self-defence or a 'real' martial art. It is also hard for the layman to see how they can offer self-defence skills against muggers and worse on the streets, since they are not overtly aggressive or offensive, which is the commonly perceived necessary component for self-defence. Both Qi Gong and Taijiquan sit oddly in the scheme of things.

Too slow for the young and too soft for the aggressively martial, Taiji's choreography is too difficult to pick up easily and its benefits are difficult to see. It is hard to package and consequently hard to sell. It has also suffered historically from infection by muddled Spiritually oriented practitioners who misunderstand its methods or principles, having studied with similarly muddled teachers. It is too cryptic for the pragmatic materialistic generation, with its talk of Qi and complex Energy theories, and too obscure for the 'weights-and-work-out' generation. Those who teach it primarily as a martial art now often neglect it as a deeper, profounder meditational and health discipline. Those who teach it for health only neglect its essential martial strategies and principles, or indeed its weapons and contact forms, thus excluding its original purpose. Those who are able to teach both aspects find difficulty in balancing the two, since generally they appeal to two different types of student.

In China, there is no such market-driven distinction and preconception. Everybody knows that Taijiquan is both martial and health giving. Good health and fitness, a balanced emotional and intellectual life is, or should be, an essential ingredient and prerequisite in martial training anyway. The need to compartmentalise and clearly label that typifies our Western culture presents no problem in Oriental culture.

The massive growth of the commercial leisure, fitness and sports market in the Western world has given rise to the high-street gym culture, as well as propelling the fashion and glossy magazine industry. It has produced a generation of fitness junkies and serial gym fanatics with the fashions, accessories, technology and an army of certified personal trainers to support it. From the 1980s aerobic craze through all the permutations of body toning, slimming routines and body beautiful, weights, stretching, postural balancing, kickbox training, Pilates and a million incarnations of Yoga, hailed as the new panacea for the beautiful and the successful, the gym culture marches on, constantly reinventing training methods and throwing up new and ultimate means of staying fit. Looking good, slim, toned and vital is the main thrust, rather than health and well-being. In all of the faddish methods that the gyms and modern health culture spawned, Taijiquan and Qi Gong terminology and principles were sometimes plundered for marketing and to add gloss and mystery to otherwise commonplace training methods.

While fewer people in China are now showing interest in investing their time in learning these disciplines, more people in the West are becoming aware and receptive to learning and benefitting from them. There is much more knowledge available now than a few years ago, and there is a growing pool of experienced and serious practitioners whose dedication to the art is building a better profile, as well as a bridge to China and the cultural roots that infuse these disciplines.

In the West there is now a great need for a comprehensive self-help health system like Qi Gong and Taijiquan but there are big hurdles, the biggest being our lack of faith in its efficacy and its culturally remote principles and theories, and our modern frenetic and pressured lifestyle. Paradoxically it is the latter hurdle that makes Qi Gong and Taijiquan so important today.

Neither discipline fits into the 'quick hit' health culture, but for those who recognise the need to do something about their physical and mental well-being and who want to make a real lifestyle choice, Qi Gong and Taijiquan are a good long-term investment.

Qi Gong and Taijiquan probably rate as the most effective and comprehensive health system available today. In addition, they offer a strategy to negotiate the trials and tribulations of our daily lives and the peaks and troughs of our happiness, and this alone may prove to be their most valuable contribution.

The downside is that learning both disciplines properly to a reasonable level can take some time, so you need to be committed and to persevere, since the benefits are cumulative. That is, the longer you do it the more you benefit. Learning the basics of Qi Gong and Taijiquan can take at least a year, and to really get inside it takes much longer. Basic Qi Gong is quick to learn, but to achieve a depth of practice can also take some time. Without perseverance and mental discipline neither Qi Gong nor Taijiquan will bear fruit.

A word of warning though: as the old Chinese saying goes, 'If you miss in the beginning by a fraction you can end up out by many miles' and be left wondering where the returns on your investment are.

Finding a knowledgeable, competent and inspirational teacher is at the root of staying with a programme until you can 'stand on your own feet'. Once you have achieved a competency in either or both disciplines, then it is yours for life. You can take it anywhere: you do not need equipment or a gym. In addition you can practise it into old age, where you will find its benefits are truly significant and possibly amazing.

Learning Qi Gong and Taijiquan is easier now than ever before with a plethora of books and teachers and organisations that can deliver good-quality study programmes. Nevertheless you still have to be motivated and persevere, and for that you need inspiration, a belief in the disciplines' efficacy and enjoyment of their beauty. Learning these disciplines is like embarking on a journey, since there will be many physical and emotional hurdles to cross. However, it remains a profound journey of self-discovery, growth and fulfilment, and that is something that makes Qi Gong and Taijiquan quite unique in modern health culture.

CHAPTER 1

Qi Gong and Taijiquan

Qi Gong

The slow, mannered movements and cryptic oriental philosophy that have defined and beleaguered a clear understanding of Qi Gong in the West for so long are only the tip of the iceberg representing a method of training and self-cultivation that must stand as one of the most, if not the most, comprehensive body–mind-oriented systems in the world.

In most parks in China, early morning is a special time when many people congregate for exercise and social interaction. It is commonplace to see large groups of people practising a variety of martial arts, including Taijiquan and also Qi Gong. Qi Gong has many faces, Taijiquan is one of them. Others can be more obscure but no less interesting. Absorbing 'Energy' (Qi) from trees and shrubs and the sun is common Qi Gong practice (Gong – achievement); holding postures, emitting different sounds, stretching in a variety of ways and moving freely in complex patterns and rhythms comprise much of the Qi Gong exercises that can be seen in the early morning. They all aim to heal, rejuvenate and invigorate the practitioners, as well as offer peace of mind and harmony in their lives.

On the streets and in the old neighbourhoods it is common to see people sitting outside their homes pressing, massaging and manipulating each other (Tui Na) or walking in slightly exaggerated or strange ways or practising a set of martially oriented movements in a slow and deliberate way. All of these activities are the common face of Taijiquan and Qi Gong in China and are an expression of an ancient traditional health culture of self-cultivation. It is based upon the belief that when our physical and energetic body is balanced, primed and harmonised with the energies of 'Heaven and Earth', we will retain our health, vigour and mental capacity well into old age. This is colloquially known as 'Eternal Spring'.

The tradition and methods of Qi Gong were undoubtedly born out of early shamanic healing and close observation of animal behaviour and natural processes and, inevitably, fear of illness, death and the apparent powers of nature. This magical-religious background was the same fertile ground from which acupuncture, herbal healing, martial arts and the Chinese indigenous religions and philosophy of Daoism sprang. Confucianism, and later Buddhism, entered the equation and contributed significantly to the flowering of Qi Gong as a system. Martial arts also became another distinct thread in the development of Qi Gong, and Qi Gong methods evolved as an adjunct to the cultivation of martial skills and power. The main aim of such practice, however, was health and healing disease, feeling in accord with the powers of nature, and cultivating a long, healthy life and even, it was believed, immortality – themes that have fascinated the Chinese since ancient times and still do.

The common term Qi Gong (Energy work) is relatively recent. In China the discipline is still sometimes referred to by its much older names, such as Yang Sheng (Nourishing Life), Dao Yin (Guiding and Inducing) and Xing Qi (Moving Breath), and these names point to the aims and methods of Qi Gong as it is commonly known today. The different terms that have been favoured over the centuries and have become associated with certain techniques and types of practice are now generally referred to as Qi Gong, an all-encompassing term for all forms and methods of practice whose aim is the achievement of 'Eternal Spring'. Under the umbrella of Qi Gong there is an enormous range of methods, styles and techniques ranging from the obscure to mainstream systems that are pretty much consistent across much of China and amongst the overseas Chinese communities. However, although the names and the forms may be generally identifiable, there are often stylistic differences and changes in emphasis. This is inevitable.

Since the founding of modern China as a communist state Qi Gong, like Taiji and many other ancient traditional aspects of Chinese culture, has undergone at first radical repression by both government and society and then acceptance, approval and development in certain areas, notably medical.

For instance, religious Qi Gong, as one might expect in a secular, communist society, has been sidelined and in some cases outlawed. However, the lines between the different strands of Qi Gong can often blur and much medical Qi Gong is by derivation Daoist and can serve both religious and medical ends. Great efforts have been made to put Qi Gong into a totally pragmatic and functional medical context stripped of any religious or mystical goals, but the goals of health and longevity are still acknowledged across Chinese society and are deeply entrenched in a health culture that owes much to Daoist Spiritual practice and influence. Although the Spiritual practice of Qi Gong is less evident in mainland China, the methods of achieving such aims are still available and are alive and well.

Martial Qi Gong has a high prominence, especially in the West, with its promise of extraordinary martial powers. It was historically developed by both Daoist and Buddhist practice and theory. However, in the West it is often taught without a proper 'counterbalance' or within an exclusively martial context. This is not conducive to a balanced result. This means that though martial ability may be improved by specific methods of Qi Gong, often the civil or personal cultivation of the individual may be neglected or even distorted in the achievement. In China the inner teachings, like the specialised Qi Gong of any martial system, were kept secret and revealed only to individuals deemed worthy of the knowledge ('indoor students'). This still continues, but the secrets are now no longer as secret and are available to many, regardless of their aims and mental readiness for such practice, on bookshelves throughout the world. In China it is understood that certain Qi Gong, if not practised properly, can cause mental disturbance and/or illness, and this is often overlooked in the Western approach to the practice of martial Qi Gong.

The Qi in Qi Gong refers on a mundane level to 'breath' or 'air', but it also relates to the idea that all life and material phenomena are expressions of a primal, unified Energy. This idea is fundamental to the traditional Chinese thinking and permeates all expressions of Chinese culture, especially medical theory and practice, martial arts, the arts and the Spiritual path. Man is considered a conglomeration of Qi, a temporary physical entity in a unified energetic field, like a wave on the sea. Our existence, life, health and functionality are dependent upon the movement, balance and abundance of that Energy, bound as our physical form and inextricably linked to a universal Energy field for the duration of our lives. Once that Energy is depleted we die and all that we are returns to the original source. Qi is the fundamental state of all material and non-material existence.

The Chinese have not traditionally tried to define Qi, accepting that it is beyond the realm of the word. Qi is generally regarded in terms of its functionality and comparative states rather than its specific properties. Like electricity, Qi is invisible but can be evidenced by its various manifestations – for example, electricity can turn a wheel or generate warmth, but we cannot see 'it'. The effects of Qi functioning define it. Pay attention to the sense of your own motion, the warmth of your body, the sense of awareness, your functional mobility, the sensation of yourself as 'living', and you are experiencing and recognising the manifestations of Qi. Chinese thinking happily attributes many functions to Qi. For instance, within the Chinese medical paradigm Qi is described paradoxically as the source of movement and movement itself. This comprises all forms of movement, from simply walking to growth, respiration and cellular activity, etc. Qi is also protective and warming, it brings about transformation, storage and distribution, and it binds and regulates our physical self. It also connects us, on a deeply fundamental level, to everything else (Yuan Qi) both coarse and subtle.

Qi Gong and medical theory further explain that there is pre-natal and post-natal Qi. Pre-natal Qi is what we are given or inherit, and post-natal Qi is what we acquire from food, air and absorption of 'Heavenly and terrestrial Qi'.

Within the body each system and organ can be described according to Qi activity/function, but also those systems and organs are holistically bound and interdependent. Currents of Qi are described as moving throughout a matrix, or web of channels (the Jing Luo and Extraordinary Channels) which penetrates the whole body and both maintains our physical integrity and optimum functionality but also links us to the energetic environment. Both cellular and molecular activity is understood as Qi activity, and so Qi is all-pervasive and the most fundamental condition of existence. Our energetic body is affected by external energetic influence and our own actiivities. Qi Gong sets out to create favourable conditions for optimising our personal 'deposit' of 'life Energy' (Qi) and to help us accumulate, generate and distribute our Qi in the body. It also teaches us to create a beneficial relationship with natural forces and conditions that can affect us positively. Qi Gong theory expresses the belief that illness is the result of Qi imbalance and can be cured by balancing our energetic disharmonies, distortions, stagnation or rebellion within us.

To do this, Qi Gong targets three key aspects: our body, our breath and our mind. It is these three that are the defining criteria of all Qi Gong practice, and all methods share in different degrees the idea that these three aspects must be 'regulated' and brought into a harmonious relationship that will benefit the whole.

Taijiquan

Taijiquan is also considered a Qi Gong, and in many instances what can be said about Qi Gong can also apply to Taiji. Taiji, considered solely as a health exercise, shares the same goals and similar methods and vocabulary of movement. However, when we come to the martial aspect of Taijiquan then there is divergence, since, although it can be said that Taiji is Qi Gong, it cannot be said that Qi Gong is Taiji. Qi Gong is not a martial art. Both disciplines, though, offer the same extraordinary health benefits.

What comprises most people's awareness of Taijiquan is the study and practice of the traditional Long Slow Form or more recently developed and easier to learn versions called short forms. In Chinese the long form is called the 'Big Slow Fist Boxing' (Da Man Quan) and is the platform on which the 'art of Taiji' is built. Whether for health or martial arts, the form is the starting point of the journey.

The building blocks or the vocabulary of the form are a number of individual martial movements, strung together with connective gestures and set into a pattern of continuous, flowing movement giving rise traditionally to 108 connected movements. The movements are derived historically from the diverse areas of indigenous Chinese martial arts, and mythologically from a fight witnessed between a crane and a snake by the originator Chan San Feng, a Daoist who supposedly marvelled at the natural, graceful and soft but deadly abilities of the two protagonists. Taijiquan, like the animals that inspired it, evolved to exhibit a sense of natural elegance, softness (disguising the hardness) and yielding in defence, while swift, accurate and hard in attack. It cultivated continuous flowing, rounded and spiralling movements to divert and neutralise an opponent's force. It advocated a calm, intuitive and naturally balanced mind, unconfused by the fight or flight instinct. Chan San Feng (the most commonly agreed founder, though possibly a mythological figure) supposedly applied Daoist ideas to existing martial structures and patterns. In this way the practice of Taijiquan came to express the universal laws of change (Yin and Yang). The achievment of understanding Yin and Yang became the achievement of the 'Dao'. In reality, it was probably much later than Chan San Feng that Taiji as a boxing art became fully underpinned by the growing sophistication of Daoist philosophy and Qi Gong theory.

Daoist insight and observation of nature, that is the Heavens, Earth and Man, formed the body of Daoist natural science, and it was this triplex unity that informed both Taiji and Qi Gong theory. Taiji and Qi Gong reflected what were considered immutable laws and natural principles, which in turn gave rise to the idea that cultivating naturalness in body and mind harmonised with nature and the prevailing conditions. The process of being 'natural' meant peeling away conditioned states and recovering a clear perceptual reality, only reacting appropriately and in accordance with immediate events. It was at once a strategy for martial engagement, a philosophy for life and a Spiritual path that brought the rewards of health, the prize of longevity and wisdom. To achieve this state was to resonate in accordance with a deeper reality, an all-pervasive, unifying principle referred to as the 'Dao'.

These ideas gave rise to specific methods of practice and training that gave Taiji its particular characteristics and which identified Taijiquan as an art concerned more with the cultivation of the 'internal' landscape and 'mindset' rather than the more 'external' physical qualities as exemplified in the Buddhist boxing systems of Shaolin. Although Taijiquan may have been created to achieve primarily martial goals, for which it was highly regarded, its Daoist roots imbued it with 'Spiritual' undertones and identified it along with Qi Gong as a path to longevity, which in Daoist culture is the reward for self-cultivation and Spiritual achievement. It is this paradoxical relationship that is at the heart of Taiji and which has undoubtedly caused such difficulty in its assimilation into Western health and martial culture, where the Spiritual and martial sit in different camps. In traditional Chinese culture there is no dichotomy here.

To achieve the methods Taiji required, and to fulfil the understanding of complementary Yin–Yang qualities like soft and hard, slow and fast, internal and external, and curved and straight, meant retraining the body, its habitual preferences and instinctive reactions and mindset. To do this, forms were practised slowly. Initially, they were probably practised as standing exercises, progressing to joined-up practice where several fixed positions may transpose into other fixed positions. The fixed positions were associated with the offensive (striking) and the transition phase associated with the defensive and changing strategies. This, however, could be applied to many martial arts if it was not for the Daoist propensity for seeing changeability as a condition of life and the idea that the hard must emerge from the soft and the soft must contain the hard and, finally, that meeting force with force was counterproductive. Indeed this contravened the profoundest universal laws of change and balance, and these concepts have engendered much misunderstanding, though they remain as true today as they probably did in the days of Chan San Feng.

The apparent non-aggression and meditative demeanour shown in Taiji is based around the concept of calm and intelligent response and strategic fighting rather than physical strength. Common perception claims attack as the best form of defence: the strongest, fastest and most aggressive will win. Taiji does not adhere to this. Instead, an opponent is encouraged to attack or commit to an attack first, defence then becomes attack and the two aspects blend into a seamless unity. Taiji theory states that in an attack fuelled by physical strength and aggressive intention, the attacker would be disadvantaged, since he had committed to action and revealed both intention and force. Taiji came to specialise in skills of receiving, diverting, neutralising and returning force. To do this, interpreting your opponent's ability, power and direction of attack was crucial. Cool, calm, skilful and empty of intention until the time arose to deliver an attack, was the preferred strategy. To achieve this mindset, slow and meditative practice and long periods holding postures (Zhan Zhuang) became the norm to retrain the body and the mind to work holistically as an intelligent whole, intuitively responsive, at once soft and yielding and then hard and penetrating.

The practitioner was expected to override muscle tension associated with the 'fight or flight' response, and to cultivate flexiblity, looseness and softness and physical and mental integration. In addition the training methods cultivated a meditative and highly alert mindset. All this paradoxically sought to increase fighting speed and effectiveness and a particular type of Energy that could be stored within the tissue of the body and issued as a force rather like a whip, or water – soft yet penetrating and awesomely powerful. This power was to remain disguised in softness, and released unexpectedly at the opponent. The energetic component is refined Qi, the trained martial Energy is Jin and the mental state is referred to as Shen. All three are intimately connected and interdependent.

The method of slowness in 'form practice' developed accuracy and allowed evaluation and interpretation of the opponent's intention and skill in practice. That slowness, however, is transformed through training strategies to achieve speed and sensitivity in real martial application.

To achieve the soft flexibility, absorbing, diverting, neutralising and sudden but fluid attacking skills, Taiji boxing cultivated a heightened awareness of postural correctness, balance and stability in one's self and then in an opponent. Taiji sought to refine the whole body to develop a kind of flexible, sustainable power, born out of the body both externally and internally moving harmoniously as a single unified force that hid its attacking ability. Hardness in attack could be manifest quickly and then returned to softness and pliability, allowing change in accordance with an opponent's attack and defence strategy. Maintaining stability in movement, whether in attack or defence, and understanding the dynamics of balance was fundamental to the training methods and fighting strategies of Taijiquan.

Being able to realise the circularity of defence that Taiji advocated meant a very sophisticated level of training and conditioning that required a high level of mental control, not only to apply the skills but to develop in conjunction internal aspects of gaining control over programmed, instinctive responses and behaviour in conflict. All of these were Daoist concepts. Since Taiji was 'of Daoism' and its methods and principles were explained by Daoist theory, it became an expression of and a path to achieving both martial and non-martial objectives, namely longevity and Spiritual cultivation. Taijiquan was a portal through which an individual could access, through long and sincere practice (Gong Fu), a permanently heightened state of 'wisdom mind', physical health, martial skills and a balanced, harmonised awareness of the ebb and flow of forces, events and turmoil that constitute life. Indeed, it was the process of martial training that revealed this to the practitioner.

The true boxer was able to discipline and cultivate himself ('virtue') and then face the onslaught of both enemy and life with equanimity ('martial'). Daoists believed that riding the waves resulted in better health and martial survival than resistance, which meant cultivating hardness and force – both of which appeared on observation finite and unsustainable. Man had a propensity to apply force against force to conquer and subdue. This behaviour was against 'nature' and steered man inexorably away from the 'true' path of the ancients, who knew that to live in harmony with nature was to find peace, happiness, prosperity and 'immortality'. Taiji became a physical manifestation of those principles, such that the practitioner resonated with the Heavenly and Earthly pulses that are the living world. In this way he achieved the 'Dao'.

Both Taiji and Qi Gong have vocabulary and ideas specific to their discipline, and it is impossible to get very far in either discipline without investigating the ideas and acquainting yourself with a vocabulary that articulates the experiences of Taiji and Qi Gong practice.

I have come across many people who have studied and practised Taijiquan for many years and they wonder, beyond the martial skills, where they are going with it. Practice should be like eating bread or rice. It is best not to have expectations, since they invariably are never fulfilled, but just to practise, listen to your body and cultivate a simple, undistracted awareness. Correct practice does bring identifiable rewards, but they are quiet and not easy to quantify. The more you practise, the more you realise that it is a deeper and profounder experience, the more mature your practice becomes. It is the evolution of these sensations that eventually allows you to become the practice and the practice becomes you. It is the practice itself that transcends purpose.

Finally, I am sometimes asked if you have to go to China or speak Chinese to understand Taiji and Qi Gong. The answer is no, but if

Taiji or Qi Gong were dishes on a menu they would taste different in China than anywhere else, even though the ingredients might be the same, and each cuisine will nourish you adequately. The Chinese approach to study and practice, however, can be significantly different from the Western approach. It would have a different emphasis and almost certainly a different timeframe. By virtue of its cultural orientation this often hints more succinctly at a 'way'. Taiji and Qi Gong are an approach to life, and the achievement of 'virtue' (De) through self-cultivation, rather than as a bit of encapsulated and acquired knowledge. It is a both a total and an informing experience.

CHAPTER 2

Nourishing Life and Eternal Spring

Since ancient times the search for longevity and immortality has been a preoccupation in Chinese culture and a major thread in Daoist natural philosophy. Daoism is the native religion of China and is commonly attributed to the writings of Lao Tze in his famously cryptic short text called *Dao De Jing* (trans. Lau 1963). Its beliefs are, however, considerably older. Nevertheless, this text stands as a seminal early work of Daoist literature. The text does not follow the rule of any methodological argument such as we might expect or wish for in the West; instead it uses parable, allegory and paradox to express the meaning and attainment of the 'Dao', the nature of which is beyond intellectual comprehension. 'Dao' means, literally, 'The Way', though its connotations are much greater.

The *Dao De Jing* formalised an older belief system based upon the idea that there is a unifying principle or Energy that permeates all material and non-material things. It is evidenced in all aspects of 'Heaven', 'Earth' and 'Man'. It is manifest in the changing nature of the phenomenal world, and the felt experience of our physical and energetic self and of our relationship to all life and the material and non-material world and beyond. Its tidal fluctuations are expressed in the theory of Yin and Yang.

Cultivating an intuitive understanding and 'tuning-in' and har-nessing this primary and universal Energy is the essential means of nourishing our life Energy and recovering an original and un-corrupted state. Recovery of this state is achieved through a long process of 'self-cultivation'. This means, in Qi Gong terms, nurtur-ing a particular and coherent physical, energetic, emotional, intel-lectual and Spiritual state. According to the *Dao De Jing* the 'way' of achievement is born out of giving up resistance, both within ourselves and our environment, and cultivating an acceptance of the natural course of events, and in turn the 'real' or 'true nature' of all things is revealed. The path of achievement results in 'virtue' (De). The virtuous person is one whose true nature is fully realised and who resonates harmoniously with the Dao. This is a person free, spontaneous, non-judgemental and deeply and intuitively connected with all that we are.

This pragmatic yet mystical text obliquely informs us that all affairs of man, nature, the Earth and the cosmos are manifestations of, and governed by, a unifying principle or Energy alluded to as Dao, which is beyond analysis and intellection. The followers of this principle became known as Daoists and their philosophy contrib-uted much to the evolution of Chinese culture.

After Lao Tze, the second most celebrated writer and thinker who added significantly to the early writings of Daoism is Chuang Tzu, whose text, known as *The Chuang Tzu* (trans. Fung 1997), ex-pounds the liberation and freedom of the individual and the spon-taneous and natural virtue of nature. It is both funny, anarchic and profound, alluding to a state whereby 'true nature' can be intuited directly. Within both the *Dao De Jing* and *The Chuang Tzu* texts it is possible to find recommendations for the cultivation of the 'virtu-ous' state (De) and health, and the prolongation of life and Spiritual enlightenment.

As great exponents of longevity, Daoists practised and studied ways of improving health by refining the body, breath and mind to achieve a harmonious and transcendent union, a spontaneous under-standing of 'true nature'. Such an elevated state, if constantly refined, could confer immortality, sainthood or sagehood. This was a blissful state, lived out in the seclusion of cloud palaces high amongst the sacred peaks of some of China's most dramatic mountain ranges. Chinese legends and paintings are full of images and characters who have achieved immortality, achieved the Dao. It is still common in households and temples alike to have statues of eight such mythological immortals whose images are enough to welcome good fortune into the house and benefit the occupier, who in turn should treat them with respect and honour their Spiritual achievements. This represents the later, more prosaic and ritualistic face of Daoist practice, which would undoubtedly have been frowned upon by the likes of Lao Tze and Chuang Tzu, who seemed to advocate a way of life unencumbered by material or Spiritual baggage.

The fascination with longevity is probably as old as man, since death and illness are realities that still haunt and frighten us. Methods to ward off illness and prolong life probably evolved from ancient practices like dance, trance-induced states and shamanic healing. Over time they must have evolved into a highly sophisticated methodology, underpinned by a theoretical foundation that was, and still is, remarkable for its holistic approach and in-depth explanation of the body as a responsive, interdependent, energetic entity that resonates in accordance with environmental conditions and indeed the bigger world. *The Huang Di Nei Jing* (*The Yellow Emperor's Classic of Medicine*; Ni 1995), dated around the third millennium BC, is still published today. It stands as the seminal text on Chinese medicine. This text, which represents the accumulated knowledge and wisdom of ancient Chinese thinking, is more than just a treatise on medicine: it is a reflection of a society whose concerns were the position of man in nature and not the dominion of man over nature. *The Yellow Emperor's Classic* describes and explains a profoundly holistic approach to the underlying cause of illness and disease and man's place in the natural world.

The traditions of Qi Gong stretch far back into antiquity, when both posture and breath control were used to heal a variety of illnesses as well as achieve longevity. Such practices revolved around the distinctly Chinese view of illness and health that was exemplified and described in *The Yellow Emperor's Classic of Medicine* and still today is significantly different from that of the West. The West was to wait a long time to achieve the same understanding and methods of treatment that were developed in China.

Along with *The Yellow Emperor's Classic on Medicine* (one of the oldest medical treatises in the world), Daoist writers and thinkers gave both substance and meaningful expression to those ancient ideas and provided the platform for a belief system that is clearly evidenced in the long thread of Chinese culture – notably painting, poetry, music, medicine and martial arts. The Daoists developed a culture of Spiritual development and self-cultivation which can still be found in modern China.

Daoists laid emphasis on living one's life 'naturally' and in accordance with natural, benign forces that shape and maintain life and harmony as observed in nature. Destructive elements harmful to the smooth passage of life seemed to be generated by humans, mismanaging affairs and out of touch with the rhythms and pulses of nature and man's true condition. For the Daoist, 're-connecting' generally meant actively disengaging from any aspect of life that created stress or wore out the body and mind prematurely, and especially misguided emperors and officials who sought to control man, society and nature.

Close observation of nature, living in a natural environment, eating natural foods and practising and developing techniques that brought the living-experience into harmony with the seasons and cycles of nature became key to the practice of nourishing life. Such practice aimed to maintain health, slow down and even reverse the ageing process and engender deep insight, wisdom and eventually physical and mental liberation. It was the wisdom of the 'ancients'. The methods, as we have inherited them, were based upon harnessing natural energies to prolong life, conserving and cultivating the 'life force' or 'vital Energy' that circulates both within us and around us, and harmonising life's passage with nature. This is the meaning of the art of 'nourishing life'. The goal is restoration, rejuvenation and 'Eternal Spring'.

Daoists believed that our bodies are a microcosm of the universe and as such blend both Heaven (cosmic) and Earth (terrestrial) energies. In favourable conditions, our bodies and minds, united and integrated, could be finely tuned and perfectly nourished by both Heavenly and Earthly energies, and by an innate capacity to achieve health and withstand illness and disease – a bit like a radio tuned in to the correct frequency. The Daoists saw the body and the mind as having both physical and metaphysical properties, and as such all the ingredients necessary to preserve and cultivate their life Energy as well as Spiritual Essence.

Qi Gong is based upon the belief that we are born with a certain potential, and that potential can be built upon and supplemented by ingesting, absorbing and cultivating Energy from outside of ourselves. A seed grown in poor soil has less chance of growing to its full, inherent potential than a seed grown in good soil and nourished by sun and rain, supplemented with fertiliser, and protected from the wind, excess heat and cold. A seed, regardless of its genetic stock, has a greater chance of realising its full potential if it is cared for properly. Our basic needs are not that different.

CHAPTER 3

Self-Cultivation and the Natural State

In the Qi Gong community Daoist teaching is considered the determining influence in the process of self-cultivation. Daoists were anti-conformist and adhered to a principle of 'leaving well alone' (Wu Wei) and non-interference. This guided personal behaviour. In the original form, they were not materialistic or acquisitional; indeed they shunned such attitudes and there are plenty of parables that reflect this position. Their ideal was of a natural order in which a social balance is spontaneously and dynamically achieved in accordance with, and responding to, the natural forces that shape the world around us, the sky above and the Earth below. Tuning in to those forces and rhythms was the key to a long and happy liberated life and a free society, unbound by ritual, dogma and rules. It was the Way of Dao.

Daoists put much emphasis on the development of the individual self as a means of returning to a pristine, uncorrupted state. Whereas Confucianism, the other great influence on Chinese society, defined and applied self-cultivation as a social tool to benefit society as a whole, Daoists sought it as a means of personal liberation.

Confucian doctrine acknowledged and blended Daoism and its ideal of 'naturalness' but abhorred its lack of interest in society and a socially relevant ideal and how to achieve it. The Daoist way was to promote the idea of self-cultivation, not in the 'acquired' and rigorous and socially engineered way of Confucianism but in a free and natural way. This could be done by the cultivation of various skills such as calligraphy, painting, poetry, music and Qi Gong. These were both a mental and a physical discipline and a portal through which an individual could achieve a physical and Spiritual resonance and a natural unification with the universal Energy.

This natural state is sometimes referred to in the Taiji and Qi Gong community as Zi Ran, 'unaffected and natural' is a term that encompasses the idea of self-cultivation and it also implies return to a pre-habitual and restored state of clear and direct intuitive perception and action. It also implies a progression, since such a state is attained through discipline, awareness, and persistent and continuous refinement.

Zi Ran implies both an achieved state and also the recovery of one that we have lost. An infant can be considered natural and intuitively intelligent and open-minded, or naturally itself. Throughout growth, however, with the acquisition of language, emotional experience and intellectual and social development, layers of connections, meaning and behaviour are laid down, enabling us to function within our society and environment. This process distorts the very natural characteristics of the individual that we so admire in children, and perhaps vaguely remember, but which become buried. It is an idea that refers to the notion of the 'uncarved block' or the analogy of the 'polished mirror'. It is an ideal born out of a philosophy of personal liberation. It looks to the natural, unself-conscious state and the 'natural' state and 'virtue' of all things.

The process of achieving 'naturalness', the 'true self', uncluttered and undistorted, the 'just-so-ness' or 'self-so-ness'(Zi Ran) of ourselves, is a process of letting go, peeling off acquired and habitual layers to reveal 'true nature' and in so doing connecting with the unifying principle. It entails the idea that through the particular (ourselves, both physical and mental) the unifying, all-pervasive principle can be felt. In achieving 'true nature' we become intuitively connected with the nature of all things and the spontaneity of change and the 'Dao'. It is an idea that can be seen in the work of Daoist-inspired brush paintings, where the intention is to reveal the intrinsic nature of the landscape, or the bamboo grove, for instance, to reveal its essential nature without undue concern for its external appearance which, after all, is the result of a conceptual and inhibiting construct layered with connotative meaning. By liberating its true nature the Dao is revealed.

Daoists believed that it was necessary to dispense with the process of defining and analysing and to dissolve the designation of subject and object, 'me' and 'it', since these create a schism that progressively removes us from our 'naturalness', our 'real self', and hence our ability to harmonise with nature. We lose our own intuitive intelligence, our early physical and mental unified sensibility of our pure state of consciousness. We lose our empathetic resonance and connectedness to the great unifying principle (Dao).

Naturalness, however, must be attained or recovered, and the process of attaining it is the aim of Qi Gong, for 'naturalness' is the preferred and most resilient state to ride out the stresses and strains of ordinary life and, crucially, to optimise our health for a longer and happier life.

The path of self-cultivation in Qi Gong terms is not what you might expect. It is in fact a letting go, a relinquishing process rather than the acquisitional one that seems more characteristic of the Western approach to self-cultivation. It is about returning to an original, clear and uncluttered state. It is also about reasserting our spontaneous acceptance of and seamless adjustment to change. It is about resting comfortably and dissolving into a simple state of being.

CHAPTER 4

Essence, Energy and Spirit

The most fundamental of all Qi Gong theories is known as the 'Three Treasures' (San Bao). This theory targets three key aspects where the work of self-cultivation must be applied if we are to nourish our life Energy. They are Essence (Jing), Vital Breath (Qi) and Spirit (Shen). On one level they are easy to understand since we all know the meaning of the words, but they can become elusive and confusing if we try to define them too precisely.

First, they are cultural constructs that articulate functional and energetic relationships. Second, as concepts they are means of orienting ourselves to the various interrelated ideas, and indeed the real sensations, that permeate and are the practice and theory of Qi Gong. Finally, and perhaps most accessible, they can be viewed on a more physiological level as sexual, generative Energy and fluids, neurotransmitters, hormones (Jing), breath/oxygen and body functionality and physical integrity (Qi), and finally emotions, intelligence/intuition, consciousness and Spirit (Shen).

The Three Treasures are the generative mobilising and consciousness potential inherent in the union of the ovum and sperm – two disparate elements bonding to spark up a life and mobilise growth. Jing, Qi and Shen propel and sustain us throughout our years, rising in a meteoric burst of Energy to maximum potential and then level-ling and slowly deteriorating towards extinction. According to the Qi Gong community, Jing, Qi and Shen are the platforms upon which we are built, and consequently the means by which we can achieve a unity of self, optimal health and longevity.

Both Jing and Shen are considered as manifestations of Qi, but at two opposite or complementary ends of the spectrum, Essence (Jing) being Yin to Spirit's Yang. Qi, though all-pervasive, is often defined by its functional relationship within us, and as such can be repeat-edly subdivided to build a picture of a web of interrelated energetic factors identified as essentially either Yin or Yang in character. This points to the essential principle that there must be a balanced state in all parts, with all interrelated elements creating a balanced, coher-ent state of the whole. Achieving that is the work of Qi Gong.

Understanding this idea of a triplex unity is complicated by the pre-birth and post-birth states. The pre-birth state can be consid-ered our genetic inheritance, whereas the post-birth state must come from ingesting food and inhaling air, as well as other 'Heavenly' and 'Terrestial' Energy. Pre-birth and post-birth Energy blend to-gether to generate the Essence, Energy and consciousness required to sustain ourselves throughout life. At one end of that 'life Energy' are the 'Essences' that generate life, growth and change, and at the other are consciousness, intellect and Spirit. When Essence, Energy or Spirit is depleted or excessive, creating an imbalance within us, then illness or death ensues.

When we are young we have an abundance of the Three Treasures. As we grow old those resources are used up and we become depleted.

The real challenge of Qi Gong is to maintain, replenish and balance the Three Treasures so that we can conserve and sustain our life Energy for as long as possible. This is Eternal Spring.

Eternal Spring does not mean to live forever, to become an immortal in the mythical Daoist sense. It does, however, mean longevity and the retention of our health and well-being, both mental and physical, for as long as we are able. In an age where we are living longer and medicine offers us so much assistance, the latter years of our lives are often accompanied by cognitive deficiency, decrepitude and mental deterioration, along with a host of diseases and conditions arising out of poor lifestyle, stress and often poor diets. Any serious discipline that sets out to improve our health with the objective of 'Eternal Spring' and longevity is worth more than its weight in gold.

CHAPTER 5

An Ordinary Life

Life is often referred to as a journey, and this is a good way of thinking about it. We all know that life must be nourished and actively nurtured so that we may grow and live a healthy, trouble-free life, for lack of proper nourishment would mean death or poor growth. Like plants to light, we naturally steer ourselves, if we can, towards resources and conditions favourable to our survival and optimal growth. This is instinctual and common to all life forms. If it is denied, the consequences can be disastrous.

At conception a process of fertilisation sparks off a remarkable process of structured growth. In Qi Gong terms, 'primal Energy' (Yuan Qi) is bound as inherited and generative information and material in the form of an egg and sperm. Their successful conjoining is the beginning of a tenuous journey of growth, maturation, deterioration and death. The egg and the sperm are often considered the most characteristic manifestation of Essence in the theory of Three Treasures. However, it is important to see them not only as physical and chemical entities, merely carriers of essential ingredients from which life grows, but as two energetic entities that conjoin to become something far greater than the parts. The combined energetic information that is our biological potential is generative Energy that propels our growth.

Our DNA as Essence is the blueprint of us as physically and mentally functioning systems. Hence it is both Essence and Energy.

Inherent within this generative Energy is the potential for consciousness, thought and intellectual development, and this is referred to as Spirit (Shen). This includes both the emotional and empathetic capacity, the directing volitional and analytical consciousness, and the higher supra-personal and transcendant mind.

Essence and Spirit are both functional aspects or manifestations of the fundamental unifying Energy or Vital Breath (Qi), the second of our Three Treasures. Qi can be considered also as the oxygen and nutrients that the mother supplies through the umbilicus to power life after conception has occurred.

The embryo forms from the fertilised egg in a structure whose growing form, developing bioelectrical, biomagnetic, biomolecular and biomechanical nature, is an expression of harnessed Energy (Qi). Within the early formation of ourselves it is our first experience and possibly our oldest memory of a unified, emergent awareness, with an as yet unwritten consciousness, a blank sheet. This first experience of our emergent 'wholeness' – cellular, liquid, material, subtle and pulsing with life Energy – remains with us in a psychosomatic sense. It is both a memory and a living awareness. At birth and in our early years, however, it is relegated to the subconscious, as functional and environmental needs come to dominate our consciousness. Nevertheless, its memory haunts us, and for some it drives them creatively to seek even in maturity the unified and undifferentiated pre-birth state. Our original unified nature and clear unwritten consciousness are the ground upon which our post-birth experiences are imprinted. It seems to me this deep memory and awareness may be the driving force of our creative human endeavours and aspirations. It is perhaps the original 'Spiritual' experience, and a deeply felt sense of the life Energy.

The first nine months in the womb are undoubtedly formative, since the growing child can sense its environment and respond to chemical and external factors. Its biological unity must be strong to prepare it for birth and survival in the external world. In Chinese traditional society the child is already considered to be aged one at birth (if it survives its first 100 days), and this is subsequently added on to the post-birth age. This seems to recognise and acknowledge the importance of prenatal life.

Birth can be either relatively easy or seriously traumatic, with many degrees in between. For both mother and child the passage from the womb to the external environment leaves an emotional and somatic imprint. The resulting imprint can affect our sense of health and general well-being, possibly for the rest of our lives. Such memories, though, get overwritten and blended into a growing sense of self as an independent and substantial volitional entity. Deep birth memories, however, lie dormant within the connective tissue of our physical self, and can influence our life experience in a negative way.

The strategies of Qi Gong access deep residual psychosomatic memories, helping us to unlock and dissolve their often debilitating effect on our adult lives.

After birth you begin to breathe independently, to nourish the body and to bring about full independent metabolic functioning. It is your first act of individuation. Inhaling air (Kong Qi) kick-starts the lungs for life as a separate entity. Mother's milk provides the essential nutrients and immunology (Qi and Jing) to nourish and sustain the infant.

The first breath is the start of a life journey that progressively evolves into independence and individuation as we move from baby to infant, to child, to teenager, to adulthood, to middle age, to old age, to death. Anything can happen on the way. We are subject to the vagaries of our genetic predisposition, our environment and a multitude of other determining factors. Maximising our survival potential is the aim of Qi Gong.

Our predisposition for coherent growth is inherent in pre-birth Jing, Qi and Shen and is reinforced by post-birth Jing, Qi and Shen, resulting from taking in food (Gu Qi) and air (Kong Qi). Solid food and water provide essential nutrients, vitamins, protein, carbohydrates, minerals and liquids, from which we metabolise essential biochemical building blocks that enable us to harvest Energy from the useful constituents of food and air. The quality and type of food we eat and the air we breathe determine the quality of our Essence and Energy (Zhen Qi). How that is transformed and distributed determines our ability to maximise our natural potential and remain free from disease and illness, and hence enjoy a long life.

We are in possession of a physiological constitution, a personal disposition, or character, and an innate intelligence. Altogether they are our potential. It is our responsibility to nourish and cultivate what we are given, but to do this these elements must be kept in optimum functional balance. In Qi Gong this is done by working on the Three Treasures, by using and enhancing our natural mobility and functionality, respiratory technique and mental cultivation.

As we grow up, we change height and shape and we refine our motor skills and our understanding of our outer and inner world. We learn to stand upright, walk, talk and function appropriately in our context. We become sexually mature and our personalities develop in complex ways. We develop emotional strategies and habits that result from our growing experiences, some healthy and some not always so healthy. Learning from our peers, parents and society we evolve and modify. Environmental, social, personal needs and pressures are all in the mix. We mature and all hope to be healthy and emotionally fulfilled as well as materially comfortable. Unfortunately it doesn't always happen that way and life can actually become a struggle, full of twists and turns, successes and failures. Our emotional lives can become knotted and muddled as a result of the blows that ordinary life can deliver. The resulting emotional landscape can leave us feeling vulnerable, stressed, sometimes anxious and often disconnected from ourselves and what is happening around us. Persistent stress is the most common condition in our modern urban society. Over a long period it reduces our natural ability to maintain our emotional and physical balance. Most of us do not have the disposition or the energetic resources for the unnatural and unrelenting pressure that we may be subject to in modern society. Indeed, in addition we often bring this stress upon ourselves through lifestyle choices, ignorance and neglect of consequences. Such consequences are likely to be life-threatening and result in debilitating illness and premature depletion of our precious resources. There comes a time when it is too hard to replenish what is too seriously depleted. Although the modern world brings enormous benefits to many, there is also a significant price to pay.

Qi Gong can play a part in maintaining an important perspective on what is conducive to our well-being, as well as constantly reasserting a balanced state and hence a more robust constitution and harmonious emotional landscape. In this way we are more able to dissolve the effects of stress and combat the wear and tear of our ordinary lives.

Life is in fact both robust and fragile and living it can be both pleasurable and difficult, but we should all be able to recognise the point where our health and well-being are compromised. In the past, decline may have been slow and gradual over a lifespan. But now there are many more factors that can bring on serious illness and premature ageing.

At a certain point we simply stop growing and often live on quite comfortably for many years. We are at a stage where our Essence (sexual Energy, sperm, eggs, and sexual and other fluids and hormonal secretions), vital Energy (sense of physical health, general well-being and Energy available for normal function and mobility) and possibly our Spirit (mental capacity and intellectual ability) seem to have passed their maximum potential and we begin to realise that we cannot do what we used to do, we are not as fit as we were, and we cannot think or act as quickly.

After a middle period of relative comfort we begin to notice our appearance changing and we become more susceptible to illness, aches and pains, and sometimes much worse. No matter how much nourishment we ingest or how congenial our environment is, we can no longer get stronger again and we begin showing the external, and feeling the internal, signs of deterioration. In addition to this natural process the cumulative effects of our lifestyle and eating habits will be catching up on us. Our personal history will be affecting our health for better or for worse, depending on how we have treated ourselves and the circumstances of our life.

Physical deterioration and possibly poor health is a wake-up call to prepare for the uncertainty of old age. Obesity, heart problems, arthritis, circulatory disorders, diabetes, stiffness and loss of flexibility, respiratory disorders and worse, cancer and other long-term degenerative disorders are all now common in our modern society. Although we are generally living much longer, the quality of our life into old age is often poor.

Informed consensus of opinion tells us that beyond the raft of normal conditions associated with age, many more conditions are brought on by a more sedentary lifestyle, poor diet, smoking and high levels of stress. Knowingly or unknowingly, we may be putting ourselves into high-risk categories. More exercise is recommended (and from an earlier age than previously). Better diet and methods for the reduction of stress all play an important part in maintaining health. Nor is it only the aged that are falling ill from lifestyle-related conditions: children are also developing conditions such as obesity and diabetes as a direct result of diet and lifestyle.

It seems our ancient biology, built for survival as hunter-gatherers in a different epoch, is vulnerable to the easy (pop into the shop and buy it rather than go out in the bush and hunt it or dig it up) availability of foods that are not particularly good for us. High in salt, fat and sugar, these foods have become staples for many children and, combined with a lack of exercise and an easier, sedentary lifestyle, prove to be dangerous to health.

Think for one minute about what you really need to keep ticking and how much Energy you as individuals burn in your lives; how much fuel you throw on the fire in order to keep it lit, and how much Energy you squander unnecessarily. When we are young we care little for such waste, since we seem to have abundant supplies, but as we get older abundance turns to scarcity and the balance shifts, often too quickly.

Qi Gong is a form of positive action that offers significant health benefits for both the young and the old. It is a window through which we can observe and impact upon our personal condition. It empowers us to assume control over ourselves and to cultivate a beneficial lifestyle that is both fulfilling and optimally healthy. It is the counterbalance to the sheer seductive weight of the modern materialistic world.

In life we have a meteoric rise, then peak, level out and slowly burn up. Unless we learn how to efficiently acquire, blend, save and nourish our Energy, and unless we oil the machine to run effectively and efficiently on less, we will deteriorate too quickly. We must start to think about our own sensation of our own life and ask ourselves if we are squandering our resources and our life Energy unnecessarily – and if we are, what can be done about it.

Age and/or illness often serve to wake us up to our mortality and we begin to seek ways of not only recovering from illness, but of increasing our chances of maintaining health and mobility and our faculties. Often it is too late, and we end up relying on medical intervention and pharmaceuticals, and this often leaves us uninvolved in our own well-being. Traditional Chinese health culture is clear that our active involvement from as early an age as possible is important. Imagine you only have a finite number of breaths in your life, preordained and written in your DNA. You can use them up quickly and inefficiently, or slowly and efficiently. Which would you prefer?

Qi Gong is the art of nourishing life through self-cultivation. It aims to conserve, replenish and rejuvenate, to maintain our health, mobility, functionality and intellectual capacity into our old age, to enable us to grow old gracefully and with dignity.

All life, however, must run its course, and eventually Energy, Essence and Spirit are so depleted that they disperse and you die.

The theory of the Three Treasures identifies the essential components of being as recognised by traditional Qi Gong communities. It is towards these components that our efforts must be targeted to increase our potential both for good health and for a longer, satisfying life. The Qi Gong community pays much attention to this theory and believes that the process of ageing can be slowed down by nourishing and conserving Essence, Vital Breath and Spirit, and by reversing the degenerative, excessive imbalances that result from living our life in an arbitrary way. Along the way Qi Gong can help us deal with illness and emotional upset, stress, and perhaps even our death.

Body, Breath and Mind

In Qi Gong terms, the body is considered as both physical (material) and energetic. Our inherited constitution and physical type are what we have to work with. There is a saying that if the hinges of a door are used regularly, they stay working properly, and if left unused, they will seize up. This basically encapsulates the strategy of body work in Qi Gong.

The body is the material aspect of the work of Qi Gong. That work generally involves movement to maintain and refine the natural functional capability of the body and its systems. Movement in Qi Gong generally means integrated, harmonious and 'soft' movement that does not build excessive strength or muscle bulk. Typical Qi Gong movement seeks to power blood and lymphatic circulation, stretch muscle, tendon, ligament and connective tissue, massage internal organs and stimulate the immune system. Qi Gong movement is not the same movement that we use in our daily lives: although the vocabulary and range of movement can be approximately the same, the manner of execution is different. Deep relaxation is the primary requirement and strategy of Qi Gong. Through deep relaxation the inhibitory tensions held deep within the muscles and tissues release energetic blockages.

Qi Gong teaches us to reduce the amount of stress and strain expended on movement and physical work (walking, running, etc.) and trains the body and mind to rest all parts that are not required for a particular task. Typically we expend far too much Energy through unnecessary tension. This is true even in the most simple of activities, like walking and even sitting. In fact we habitually over-expend, and studying how to deal with this and developing 'relaxed' and 'appropriate' movement and Energy awareness is the first level of Qi Gong (Fang Song Gong). It is achieved through learning body alignment in both stationary positions and complex co-ordinated movement. Achieving this is a considerable feat in itself and applying it across all the activities of our daily life requires us to maintain body awareness until we can recondition ourselves physically to undertake ordinary tasks with the minimum of Energy expenditure.

Once we have achieved a certain level of relaxed mobility, we can then start to develop awareness of our energetic self. Relaxed movement increases our flexibility, over time, and a naturally elastic strength emerges, bringing a new sense of our physical nature as a more integrated and harmonious whole, rather than a mechanical system of parts. Cultivating the sense of our body both externally and internally opens the door for a closer investigation and integration of our gross and subtle physical and energetic levels.

Awareness grows as practice of Qi Gong progresses, and so does the accompanying sense that the body comprises an energetic web that permeates and wraps around us. That Energy has movement and flow, and disharmonies, blockages, stagnation and rebellion become real sensations. Cultivating the smooth and unhindered flow of Energy throughout and around the body is a main objective of Qi Gong and is the key to achieving optimum health and mental well-being.

In addition to the body work, we also need to bring respiration into the equation. This is the post-birth breath that brings that crucial component of air, oxygen (Qi) into our bodies to give and maintain life. The correct manner of achieving respiratory efficiency is discussed later on, but suffice it to say that most of us have poor respiratory technique and this can have a major impact on our health. In Qi Gong when we talk about breath and respiration, we mean refining the whole process of diaphragmatic movement and an optimised posture and muscle usage to power efficient respiration to achieve adequate oxygenation and gaseous exchange. We also mean refining respiration with functionality.

Respiration is both volitional and autonomic, and as such provides us with a functional link between our external and our internal environment that we can train. It is a link that allows us to affect our internal landscape, at the deepest level of our physiological, mental and energetic self. In Qi Gong, respiration is the key to Energy cultivation and accumulation. By harmonising breath with movement, Energy can be controlled and mobilised.

When the body is relaxed, inhalation and exhalation seem to be a total, unimpeded and complete body experience. From foot to head to hands, our whole body seems to breathe. The rhythmic inhalation and exhalation are accompanied by sensations of internal movement which we can call 'energetic movement'. On inhalation, for instance, the body seems to compress and 'condense' Energy at its centre (Dan Tian) and into the bones, while on exhalation it feels energetically expansive, flowing out from the centre to the skin and extremities. This is a physical sensation. In the practice of Qi Gong movement we quickly realise that harmonising breath and relaxed movement changes the sensation of movement favourably and enhances not just the functionality of movement but the quality of the felt experience.

As Energy is modestly expended we feel an accompanying replenishment. Combined specific physical movement and harmonised respiration optimise the release and distribution of energetic resources within the body, not just acting on and within the area of movement, but across the whole internal landscape, affecting and activating organs and muscles alike, while related areas of the body rebalance to accomodate those movements and use of energetic resources. In this way movement can be used to activate and tonify deep internal organs and glands, as well as to 'draw' Energy by replenishment of specific areas. This is an important aspect of Qi Gong for healing and health maintenance.

The mechanism and chemistry of breath not only facilitate all metabolic functions but also allow us to sense and adjust the ebb and flow of our energetic tide, linked to our biological rhythm and our emotional condition and environmental stress. Breath is a mechanism which allows us to harmonise body function, increase vitality, health and mental well-being. Breath reflects both how we feel emotionally and how we respond to circumstances.

Conversely, by bringing breathing under control through Qi Gong training, we can use it to impact favourably on our emotional and environmental stress response. Cultivating our respiratory technique enables us to regulate the critical and influential physiological and emotional processes, thus cultivating our health and well-being and nourishing our life Energy.

Both movement and respiratory techniques are used to cultivate and accumulate Energy (Qi) and mobilise and distribute it. Correct technique allows the body to purge excess or replenish deficiency, as well as promote free and unhindered circulation and abundance. When this is achieved it is most commonly observed in the quality of integrated and harmonious movement.

The last of the Three Treasures is 'Spirit' or mind (Shen) and it is the most important of all. However, this is only realised when you have made some progress on developing the first two. Essence and Energy, cultivated respectively as body and respiratory technique, are both necessary to maintain life and to support and nourish not only the functions of life, but also the higher levels of consciousness. From emotional 'heart/mind' (Xin) to the volitional mind, the mind of the will, and ideas and meaning (Yi), Spirit (Shen) encompasses all aspects of mental activity and consciousness. In Daoism it is also equated with a 'soul' or 'Spirit' in the sense of an entity that can separate itself from the body at death. Commonly Shen Qi is the term given to the vital principle as evidenced in the sense and appearance of vitality and mental force in a person.

The Qi Gong community believes that Shen is an energetic state that can be enhanced by certain physical and mental strategies and techniques. As an energetic state, Shen is reinforced and elevated by the activities of Qi Gong. As Energy is accumulated and mobilised and the body's physical and emotional balance is fine-tuned, the Shen can be purified, like rainwater filtering through rock. The process purifies. The end result is a heightened state of clarity and awareness and a return to a natural and intuitive mindset. As a state of mind this can be likened to a Spiritual awakening.

The process of cultivating Shen is a process that can be considered as meditative. Qi Gong practice requires the individual to focus the mind in a meditative way, where the object of that meditation or mental focus might be, for instance, internal sensations on one of three Dan Tian (upper, middle and lower Energy centres) or establishing connective currents between different parts of the body, or simply dissolving tension or cultivating breath and body awareness. To do this successfully, the mind must inhibit its mischievous 'monkey' nature and the 'internal dialogue' must be stilled. This is an enormous challenge, but the success of Qi Gong is directly related to this acquired ability and the psychosomatic state that it engenders. By inhibiting the brain 'chatter' associated with the activities of the cerebral cortex, the autonomic nervous system switches from the stress-related 'fight or flight' mode of the sympathetic branch to the restorative mode of the parasympathetic branch. This, of course, is one of the crucial keys to the restorative and healing benefits of Qi Gong. It is also the key to a deeper awareness of the fundamental nature of consciousness and 'Spiritual' achievement.

Some Qi Gong practice concentrates more on cultivating the breath and Spiritual aspects of Qi Gong but tradition regards the body work as important groundwork to create the right physical and energetic conditions for Spiritual development.

Qi Gong's aims are holistic in that it works on the belief that the whole is primary and is greater than the sum of parts. The mind, respiration and the body, therefore, should all be worked on together until each aspect is regulated and harmonised. The three elements of the Three Treasures feed each other in an upward direction, but the downward direction must also be implemented throughout practice. This means that the guiding, inducing and regulating force of the mind must be brought to bear over a prolonged period of practice to regulate/control the body and the breath in particular ways. As the body is refined and brought to a deeply relaxed state, the sense of its energetic qualities is revealed and awareness grows of our energetic self and how we acquire, accumulate and distribute our Energy. It is one of the difficulties and paradoxes of Qi Gong that we need to observe and direct ourselves from top-down to cultivate the bottom-up relationship.

The benefits of Qi Gong are directly related to the mind's ability to engage and solve the physical and intellectual puzzle that Qi Gong often seems to be.

Truly refined Shen is associated with an 'enlightened' Spiritual state, sometimes referred to as 'returning Shen to void'. It is the end result of a long process of self-cultivation and nourishment. The Spiritually charged stage of Shen implies a 'pre-anything', undifferentiated ground, without subject or object, at ease with prevailing conditions, emotionally balanced and behaving accordingly to conserve and restore ourselves. In Qi Gong this mode of behaviour is often referred to 'Wu Wei', sometimes translated as 'non-volitional action', and sometimes as 'achieving the Dao'. It is both the result of practice and the aim of practice. It implies a deeper, intuited understanding of all processes and of our human condition and energetic state, as well as of the laws of change as reflected in the theory of Yin–Yang. Shen can also refer to the inscrutable actions of Yin and Yang and imply that understanding, or giving up resisting change, is the state of Wu Wei – the result of harmonising ourselves with the deep conditions that govern life and, in turn, our own health and well-being.

Shen can also be considered as a transcendent state devoid of mental constructs, repulsion and attraction, the subject and the object of our rational and conceptualising mind. It is believed that the achievement of such a state confers longevity and, in mythological terms, 'immortality' and the wisdom of the sage.

Ordinarily, however, Shen can be experienced as a varying mental tension and an awareness of our living conscious vitality. We are all capable of it and we can all 'do it' but, like our body and our breath, we take it for granted and generally only exercise the force of the mind in the service of our material needs. Qi Gong harnesses mental power and uses it to train the body, train the breath and finally, in so doing, trains mental power itself. It is a remarkable and circular process.

Firming the Shen is training the mind in Qi Gong terms. This is an important aspect of Qi Gong and is usually considered as having two aspects: Xin (heart, moral nature, emotional mind and intention) and Yi (will, ideas, intellect and volition). In Qi Gong, Yi Nian is the most commonly used term, and refers to the formed idea or thought and its application to movement, either physical or energetic. The difficulty is that both must be employed in cultivating the Shen. Both must be nurtured throughout practice, eventually achieving a more and more subtle blend and refined emotional and volitional awareness and guiding intelligence of Xin and Yi.

It is the combined sensory and emotional awareness, intention and directing will or idea that in the beginning of Qi Gong directs movement and functionality. Body work and training integrated respiratory technique must both come under the direction of mental intention (Yi Nian) or will. The sensations (Xin) of energetic accumulation and internal movement that are cultivated in Qi Gong can be directed by mental focus as well. Indeed the directing thought, the idea, can be thought of as Shen inducing Qi. By placing the mind's attention at a particular place on the body, the sensation and energetic value of that place can be altered. By tracing a course within, or on the body, a connectivity can be established, a path or current can be created. Over a prolonged period of practice, definite beneficial sensations of internal energetic movement can be felt, like currents in the sea, and their effects understood. This ability is important in the art of Qi Gong healing, where the practitioner's Qi can be directed into the patient to mobilise, tone, purge and favourably distribute their Energy to 'balance' them.

The Shen can be cultivated for Spiritual, medical or martial ends. The most important point to remember, however, is that the Shen grows and is fed by the energetic properties cultivated in Qi Gong. It is refined through practice and meditation. It is the mental harmony that settles the potentially disturbing emotional mind. Qi Gong practice can lead to higher and higher refinement, until all the strategies and methods dissolve and a high level of skill and control becomes a subtle mental and Spiritual achievement.

Each element of this Triplex Unity (Three Treasures) is a part of the whole, and each part is activated and cultivated in a process of study. Their value dawns through that process, and their interdependent meaning and workings becomes clear. The cultivation of Shen, however, remains the crowning glory of that process and is the goal and the highest achievement we can aspire to. It is both a deep and connected sense of our living self, and a transcendent sense of a consciousness unbounded. It is both personal, mundane and universal.

CHAPTER 7

Stillness and Movement

The theory of Taiji explains the generation of two complementary, yet apparently opposing states known as Yin and Yang. This is not the theory of Taiji boxing yet, but the metaphysical theory that articulates a model for describing the nature and processes of the material world, universe and beyond. In particular it seeks to describe the processes of stillness and movement, emergence and deterioration, excess and depletion. It alludes to the apparently anomolous nature of the material world, and specifically to the interrelated nature of those apparently opposing states. It is this theory that has lent its name to Taijiquan, 'the boxing art'. It is a theory that states that all things are inherently unstable but seek dynamic equilibrium, and that all things are essentially impermanent and subject to continual change.

Taiji as a metaphysical theory is synonymous with the Dao expounded by the indigenous Chinese religion and natural philosophy of Daoism. The Dao alludes to both a fundamental unifying Energy (Qi) and the governing laws of nature expressed in terms of Yin or Yang. The action of the Dao can be intuited through understanding change, which is the fundamental characteristic of the material/phenomenal world. In the distant past, Chinese thinkers believed that the underlying unity and the laws that governed change could be deciphered and understood through divination (regarding which, see the divinatory text the I Ching, (*Book of Changes*) (Wilhelm 1965), and perceived intuitively through reflection and contemplation, or through a process of self-cultivation and empathetic understanding.

The Dao, expressed as natural laws, events and their processes, and Qi, as the fundamental and unifying Energy, underpin many aspects of traditional Chinese culture and thinking. Cultivating personal Qi to harmonise with natural laws and forces that govern man and nature became an endeavour in Chinese culture, since to 'achieve the Dao' was to achieve a state of transcendent connectivity to the Heavenly and terrestrial powers, and thus the ability to be in tune with the governing factors of nature and the events of man. Longevity and possibly 'immortality' were associated with the wisdom and refined physical state accrued by those wise practitioners.

According to the Chinese way of describing the emergence of matter, all substance and material reality emerged from the cosmic primordial condition referred to as Wu Ji, commonly called 'the One'. The One is the Dao, the void, the source, or that which existed before the universe; the fundamental and underlying energetic reality of all existence. It is from this state that Yin and Yang, 'the two' emerged, and so, consequently, did the myriad things that constitute our physical world. (See the *Dao De Jing* by Lao Tze (trans. Lau 1963).)

Yin and Yang are present in all aspects of our substantial (material) and insubstantial (energetic) world. Typified by change, the two complementary states of stillness (Jing) and movement (Dong) are evidence of the Dao, just as shadow is the evidence of light (the sun). Other obvious changing states like dark and light, down and up, empty and full, growth and depletion, which in Western science may be considered as opposite states, were seen by the Chinese as evidence of the Dao and could be described in terms of Yin and Yang or degrees of either one or the other. Yin and Yang were therefore considered as manifestations of the same fundamental energetic state referred to as Taiji (Dao), apparently both opposite and inherently complementary. Each state is a condition of the other, and they exist simultaneously in a dynamic balancing act.

According to Taiji theory, all phenomena therefore express the existence of a fundamental Energy (Qi) that permeates and constitutes everything. All natural phenomena point to it. While in their balanced state (Taiji) Yin and Yang remain unified, equal and 'still', inherent in them is the propensity for change and separation or 'movement'. Stillness and movement bring about change, and change is the defining characteristic of the material/phenomenal and natural world. Maintaining the balanced state within the context of change is the process of life itself, and excess or deficiency in that balancing act will cause an imbalance which, if not corrected, will bring about the collapse or degradation of any particular state, system or process.

The challenge of Qi Gong is to bring about and maintain a harmonious dynamic balance of Yin and Yang qualities within ourselves and within the bigger context of our environment.

According to the theory, the Taiji continues to generate further states of increasing complexity and interrelated systems in accordance with its inherent potential for change. Evidence of this state of Taiji or the Dao can be seen in all aspects of the physical world, whether microcosmic or cosmic, all of which are in constant flux by virtue of their interdependence and reciprocal influence.

Early Chinese thinkers expressed this view succinctly in the I Ching (*Book of Changes*; Wilhelm 1965), a divinatory text describing the attributes of 64 conditions arising from the interdependent play of Yin and Yang. Change is considered an immutable principle or a law of nature. Understanding true nature and the principle of change was a key to understanding the nature of all events and things and the ways of man, Heaven and Earth. The highest achievement was, and is, to gain insight into nature by cultivating a perfectly balanced and refined state within the changing context of ourselves and our life condition, resonating with the deep universal pulse and unifying principle. This awareness leads inexorably to an intuition of a void state as the source, or Wu Ji.

The state of Taiji is beautifully and succinctly illustrated in the diagram of the Two Circling Fish (see below), while the empty circle would illustrate the state of Wu Ji. This extraordinarily significant Yin–Yang symbol has become iconic in popular culture and its deeper metaphysical meaning has consequently suffered degradation, but, like the symbol of the Cross, it is one of the most powerfully charged and mystical symbols in the world. It points towards a simple and profound philosophy and experiential truth as well as a pragmatic strategy for life.

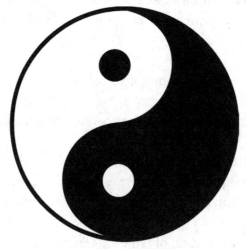

Figure: Two circling fish, Yin-Yang, Taiji Diagram

Beyond the state of undifferentiated unity representing perfect harmony and the Taiji (Dao), the symbol also graphically illustrates how a condition or a state moves inexorably to a point that has predominantly Yin or Yang attributes, from which its complementary state must eventually emerge, since one state is a condition of the other. The process is continuous and universally applicable. Whether it takes a millennium or a day or a moment makes no difference, no matter whether it refers to cosmic disturbance, the movement of the moon, tidal flow or the world of microorganisms. It is all interrelated, endlessly emergent and changing. The diagram therefore cleverly illustates how emergence and depletion are harmonised to retain a state of perfect balance within change. Holistic balance is therefore actively sought and cultivated in the practice of Qi Gong, and as such it capitalises on the inherent homeostatic nature of living organisms and natural systems.

Change is a condition that we witness in all the phenomena that comprise our material world and our experience of it and ourselves. According to Taiji theory, change is the oscillation between both movement and stillness, two opposite but complementary aspects of the Taiji (Dao). Stillness is inherent in movement, and movement in stillness. Stillness is considered the mother of movement. It is understanding these two aspects that provides the strategy for cultivating the balanced state that is the goal of Qi Gong and the theoretical basis for Taijiquan as a boxing art.

Qi Gong starts with outside movement, inside stillness, progressing to outside stillness and inside movement. This is internal Energy moving like currents under a still ocean.

The terms of Yin and Yang are the language of Dao, and refer to our world in both energetic and functional terms. Everything is Energy. It is simultaneously both nothing and something, particle and wave, visible and invisible, emergent and dispersing, dependent and independent, still and moving. Accordingly all life, all material systems, inherently seek balance in relationship to themselves and their environment. As such, life and the phenomenal world appear as harmonious and self-sustaining, giving the appearance and feeling of a permanent continuous state. We lend concrete value to this supposed permanence in our conceptual thinking, language and culture, yet it is ceaselessly changing and essentially impermanent, having no real foundation in itself.

Within our body and mind, which are the primary realm of Qi Gong practice, we can utilise stillness and movement as a strategic approach to restoring, enhancing and maintaining balance within the context of our own internal systems and the external environment. This is both the Way of Dao and the achievement of Qi Gong and Taijiquan.

CHAPTER 8

The Small Universe

Our own physical and mental world also manifests in ways that are described as Yin and Yang. This means of describing states and degrees of well-being and health is based upon the idea that man is a small universe, both contained and inextricably linked to the environment. Man is a microcosm of Heaven and Earth and is subject to the interplay of cosmic and terrestrial energetic forces, with the Heavens as Yang (not meant here in any religious context) above us, and below us the Earth as Yin. We stand vertically in a polarity that connects the two, in the way that a lightning rod connects electrical Energy in the atmosphere to the Earth. Man therefore shares in the interplay of both cosmic and terrestrial energies. The combined and blended energies within us are constantly being informed, balanced and influenced by our relationship to both what is above us and what is below us, and also by our immediate environment. Although we are a self-balancing system, we are constantly being influenced by unseen forces around us.

As physical and mental entities we have our own internal climate and landscape that must function both to keep our life systems working as well as to connect us with the cosmic and terrestial world that surrounds us. Internally and physically we are a landscape of organs, muscles, blood, bone, fluids, tissue, etc., all of which exhibit both Yin and Yang qualities, although they are generally identified functionally as having predominantly either one or the other orientation. As such, the internal world must constantly seek physiological balance (homoeostasis) within itself and in the external environment. Within every system and sub-system there is the potential for imbalance resulting from changing conditions within us and without. This produces a state of either depletion or excess, thanks to a multitude of causal factors, many environmental, some genetic, some pathogenic, and many resulting from lifestyle.

We are always subject to influence by either adverse or benign conditions. Similarly, our mental and emotional landscapes are always susceptible to disturbance, which in turn can impact upon the balancing act that is entailed in the equilibrium of our physical and energetic self.

The needs and actions of man often run contrary to the natural and harmonious relationships of Yin and Yang and the way of the Dao. Taiji and Qi Gong place great emphasis on understanding the interplay between energetic shifts in the body and facilitate proper adjustment to constantly changing conditions.

Qi Gong as a discipline and art cultivates behaviour and methods of movement and a mindset that promotes the balance within change that is symbolised by the Taiji diagram (see page 66).

In Taiji boxing and Qi Gong, stillness is associated with Yin, and movement with Yang. Without one there cannot be the other. Stillness is considered the origin of movement. Movement must always return to stillness, since it is unsustainable. Within movement (Yang), however, there is also stillness (Yin) as a precondition of movement. For example, the extreme physical work of a long-distance runner is Yang, but internally the mental component of will and endurance may be considered Yin. Such components may be subdivided. It all depends on the frame of reference.

The strategies of Qi Gong are based upon understanding this fulcrum of change and the degrees of change. Qi Gong aims to generate movement from stillness and stillness in movement. Movement requires the practitioner's centre of balance and centre of sensation and responses to be united and still, since it is from the undistracted stillness that thought guides responsive movement. Even within movement the centre must remain still. Think of a bowl with a ball in the centre. The ball finds this centre naturally by dint of gravity. If the bowl is tipped, the ball will roll off the centre, causing the bowl to tip further; if it is tipped back too quickly, the ball will roll to the opposite side, unable to regain the centre. If the bowl is pulled or pushed quickly, the ball will not move at the same speed as the bowl and will be thrown off centre and left behind. If, however, the bowl is kept horizontal and even and the movement is calm, accelerating evenly and smoothly with no excess force allowed to impact on it, the ball will remain central and unmoved. This sense of a still centre is crucial to establish. It comes from both postural adjustment and trained skill, and from fixing attention on the centre. At some point, of course, the bowl and ball metaphor needs to be discarded because single-pointed focus generates a still mind, which in turn promotes awareness of, and command over, the still centre, the fulcrum of mobility. Through practice, this become a pyschosomatic fulcrum, which means the body is integrated with the will of the mind, unimpeded by a dislocation between the physical and the mental. Both Taijiquan and Qi Gong require the student to cultivate an awareness of stillness and movement. That is finding and 'firming' the centre as well as understanding how it both generates movement and functions within movement.

Refining both is a long process, and in that process there are thresholds of awareness and hurdles to jump. Refinement is the result of practising Qi Gong and adjusting the Small Universe so that harmonising ourselves between Heaven and Earth becomes an experiential reality, and not just an intellectual exercise or a physical challenge.

CHAPTER 9

Disharmony – Thieves, Hooligans, External Influences and Common Sense

Our lives are punctuated by emotional and physical events, some good, some bad, some great, some small. Many affect us deeply, but we move on, and we often excise the unpleasant and trivial ones from our conscious mind or assign them to a shelf in our memories without much concern for how those events may have impacted upon our mental and physical well-being. Big life events like love, divorce, births (including our own), injury, illness and death can have a strong and lasting impact upon us. Such events and their resulting emotions can colour our subsequent emotional well-being, our behaviour and our physical health.

Traditional Chinese health culture has always understood that life's events and their emotional impact are significant factors in our health and illness. Its premise is that our life is a conglomeration of Energy (Qi) whose sustainability is dependent on certain factors.

Optimal balancing and conservation of Energy resources is crucial if we are to live out our lifespan in reasonably good physical and mental health. Depletion or damage to those resources will quickly bring about illness or death.

Depletion over time, however, is a natural process and the practice of Qi Gong aims to enhance and prolong the normal lifespan by maintaining a perfect dynamic balance for as long as possible. Specifically, this means both to conserve and replenish, and to distil our energetic resources and distribute them appropriately. Optimal health, renewed vigour and possibly longevity should follow. In the business of self-cultivation (Qi Gong), conservation is very important. The senses of sight, sound, taste, smell, touch, and in addition talking and thinking — are all considered activities that can deplete natural vitality or Energy and possibly harm our energetic resources and their functional ability. Anyone on the path of self-cultivation must therefore pay great attention to this. Closing down the sensory impact on mental activity is considered a mode of Energy conservation. The senses are described in Qi Gong society as 'thieves', and with good reason when you consider the life-long profusion of sensory stimuli and the sensory overload we subject ourselves to with television, the computer, reading, and our sensory engagement with our general surroundings. It becomes easy to understand how our Energy can become depleted. Excessive exposure to, or indulgence in, sensory experiences is considered harmful to our vital Energy. It can bring about confusion, indecision, lack of vigour, depression and anger. Periods of focusing our awareness internally, 'forgetting' the exterior world and thereby enhancing the body's internal restorative ability, are considered important aspects of self-cultivation that bring about favourable conditions for nourishing 'life Energy'.

It is common for us to become addicted to a high level of mental stimulation created by our sensory connection to the environment. If we do not get this we may feel bored, unstimulated and depressed. It is for these reasons that the senses are sometimes called thieves, since, while the senses feed our mental faculties and provide the information for the story that is ourselves, they can also deprive us of our well-being and equanimity. Through the senses we follow our preferences and negotiate our way through the world. Sensory information feeds and colours our emotional world, and how our mind interprets and deals with those emotions can play a determining role in our physical and mental health.

Beyond excess sensory exposure, events that surround us can also impact upon our health and can put enormous strain on our sense of vitality. For instance, pressure from work, a difficult relationship or a death may stress us emotionally and physically and deplete our resources and sense of vitality and well-being. Even a slight shock or an emotionally charged incident may leave an awkward residue of emotional disturbance. This may happen to us over a prolonged period or it may be sudden and overwhelming.

According to Qi Gong theory, excess emotions deplete and disperse our vital Energy, and for this reasons they are referred to as 'hooligans'. These are not the everyday emotions that give rich content and texture to our lives, but an excessive or inadequate level of emotion compared to what is appropriate to an event. Nobody would dispute the importance of emotions and their role in individual wellbeing and the affairs of man as a whole, but at times we need to be able to dissipate difficult and strong feelings which arise in response to events around us.

Qi Gong and traditional Chinese medicine identify seven key emotions that impact on our health and emotional well-being. They are: joy, anger, sadness, grief, anxiety, fear and fright. These are more generally and conveniently referred to in Qi Gong as *five* emotions: joy, anger, sadness, anxiety and fear. All these emotions are natural. We feel them often, sometimes daily. But excess in the form of prolonged or sudden overwhelming emotion can precipitate an energetic imbalance which in turn can precipitate illness or disease.

Each emotion is energetically associated with an organ in the body: joy with the heart, anger with the liver, sadness with the lungs, anxiety with the spleen and fear with the kidneys. Described by function, these five organs (considered primarily as Yin (Wu Zhang) organs) produce, transform, regulate and store Energy, and as such their maintainance is vital to good health. Qi Gong pays much attention to regulating and balancing these organs, and there are Qi Gong forms that are totally devoted to this.

Since it is considered that emotions may unbalance the internal climate, it follows, conversely, that any imbalance in an organ may precipitate emotional imbalance. For instance, anger may affect the liver, but an imbalanced liver may induce anger.

Self-cultivation through Qi Gong therefore requires that great care be taken in guarding the 'outflow' of Energy resulting from too much sensory input, and much attention must be paid to calming excessive emotions so as to preserve the balance of the organs and internal mental climate.

In addition, traditional Chinese doctors and Qi Gong masters alike typically warn against other conditions that can bring about degeneration and loss of vital Energy. Fame, avarice, gluttony, deceit and envy, as well as excessive sexual activity are all considered to be dangers and induce destructive excess (see Wang and Moffet, 1994, p.16). This pretty much precludes vast areas of Western popular culture, personal ambition and hedonistic behaviour. Most religions have a similar view, though their stance is more moral than the Daoist view, which concentrates primarily on conservation of Energy.

Our habits and actions create webs of complication in our lives that consume us, literally overloading, depleting and distorting our energetic resources and making it difficult for us to maintain a reasonable and optimum balance as well as a clear mind. As any trapeze artist knows, distraction or uneven weighting makes staying on the tightrope doubly difficult.

Although we are well equipped to balance ourselves to accomodate certain levels of stress, the persistence of circumstances that cause us extreme emotional and/or physical stress will bring about overload and system damage – or worse, failure.

In addition to internal imbalance brought on by strong emotions or inordinately compelling needs and ambitions, we are also subject to invasion by what are called the six 'external pernicious influences'. These are environmental factors that may jeopardise the energetic balance of the body, and include wind, cold, fire heat, dampness, dryness and summer heat.

Most of us are aware that weather conditions can disturb us; we have probably all felt the annoying effects of cold or wind or heat on and in our bodies, and indeed our mental states. We commonly speak of cold and damp 'getting inside' us and precipitating our yearly colds and flu.

Anyone who has lived in China or in extreme climates will know something of this, and will definitely understand why it is so important to guard against these climatic and seasonal patterns. In Beijing, for instance, the summer can be very hot and dry, almost desert-like, whereas in the winter the winds are strong, bone-dry, and the temperature could be -14C. Both conditions are extreme. In Guangzhou in the far south the summers are very hot and humid and the winters can be chilly and very wet. The weather is considered a serious factor to be reckoned with and hence the preoccupation in Chinese medicine and Qi Gong practice with warding off the stressful effects of these six pernicious influences on the body's systems. Avoid Qi Gong practice in windy conditions, over-exposure to the sun, damp and cold places. It is mostly common sense, really, and we were all brought up to pay attention to dressing appropriately and protecting ourselves from the weather and its effects.

Qi Gong seeks to strengthen the body to build protective Energy (Wei Qi or Guardian Qi) which guards us from the penetrating influence of those climatic conditions, and to maximise our capacity for resistance. Although the pernicious influences are not pathogenic in themselves, they can weaken certain organs and our defensive systems, which in turn can create the conditions for pathogens to invade.

Within the overall art of Qi Gong and the business of self-cultivation and nourishing our 'life Energy', awareness of the depleting and damaging effect of the senses, emotions and environmental conditions is important, since the aim of Nourishing Life (Yang Sheng i.e. Qi Gong) is to guard against loss and balance all areas of physiological and emotional activity so as not to deplete Essence, Energy or Spirit.

CHAPTER 10

Cultivating Energy

Difficulties

Traditional Chinese doctors address the business of healing and preventing illness by balancing, mobilising and distributing the body's Energy with acupuncture, herbal medicine, massage and other methods. Qi Gong is one of those methods. However, you do not need to be trained in Chinese medicine to practise Qi Gong (though an understanding of the principal ideas helps if you are to go deeply into the subject). What is more important for the student is to have an open and attentive mind, for it is the experiences that Qi Gong offers that are most important.

The traditional methods of healing work on the relative energetic states described as conditions pertaining to 'excess' or 'deficiency' within the functional systems of the body. Chinese medicine has evolved methods of treatment for optimising biological functionality by targeting different areas on the energetic map of the body so as to balance these states and redistribute Energy.

However, amongst the healing systems that comprise traditional medicine in China, Qi Gong stands alone as possibly the oldest and the most comprehensive, since it can be practised alone, without any intervention from another. It can also increase the value and effectiveness of acupuncture and acupressure or medical massage (Tui Na) when incorporated into those methods. Medical Qi Gong has also developed Qi emission therapy, where an experienced practitioner can direct his own Energy at or into another person to beneficially affect energetic imbalance, and tone and/or purge and redistribute the patient's Energy. It is a method widely used in China. In the Western healing traditions it probably equates most closely to the idea of 'healing hands'. Regular Qi Gong practice is both prophylactic and tonifying, giving us the best opportunity to avoid illness. Just as we say 'an apple a day keeps the doctor away', the same can be said of Qi Gong, only perhaps with more conviction.

Our energetic currents and paths have been well mapped over millennia by Chinese scholars. Their mapping identifies a system of interconnected energetic streams and reservoirs that run throughout the body, surfacing at various points on the body and binding within a symmetrical matrix. They do not seem to have material substance in the way that the vascular, lymphatic or nervous system has. Yet when manipulated or stimulated, these Jing Luo ('channels') can adjust the effective functioning of our internal system in both a general and a specific way, and also our ability to protect ourselves from adverse environmental factors and pathogens as well as facilitate our own healing, self-balancing potential.

In China this idea is part of the daily fabric and health culture, so the use of Qi Gong as a means of stimulating and adjusting the 'Energy values' and Energy distribution throughout the body to improve and maintain health requires no cultural adjustment or leap of faith. Acceptance of the idea of Qi can be a fundamental difficulty for Qi Gong practice in the West, and is a major hurdle in accepting Qi Gong as a valid health system for anyone whose culture rejects the veracity of the original premise.

Entering the 'gate' of Qi Gong requires an open mind, since it is possible to build and refine an awareness of ourselves that equates to the idea of Qi and the theories of Chinese medicine. There is currently no other model available to us that can articulate the effects, awarenesses and sensations that evolve from the practice of Qi Gong.

On this basis, some Qi Gong sets and forms are easier to practise because they have clear external (physical movement) characteristics that sit more comfortably within the commonly perceived dualistic and mechanistic view of our mind and body that is prevalent in Western cultures. Qi Gong is most accessible at this level, but at some point anyone interested in pursuing Qi Gong further and nourishing life through self-cultivation must become familiar with the root ideas, and more refined in their practice, as their experience of Qi Gong develops.

On a simple level, Qi Gong is designed to relieve us of excessive mechanical 'stress and strain' and to ensure optimal functioning. On a deeper level it beneficially affects the functioning and the tone of the main organs and critical systems and processes of our body. On yet a deeper level Qi Gong cultivates and refines the sense and functioning of our energetic body and its relationship to mental activity and the environmental energetic conditions. Further practice brings about a balancing and calming of habitual emotional response and a growing sense of internal stillness. Beyond this lie the meditational achievements of a deep stillness from which thoughts arise and dissolve and we sense the pure, undifferentiated field of consciousness that is our original state of being. There are many hurdles along the way to achieving these levels of Qi Gong.

All Qi Gong relies upon the cumulative effect of regular and sustained practice over a long period of time (Gong Fu). The achievement of Qi Gong, however, necessitates correct methods and practice, and correct mindset in practice and daily life if we are to bring about positive, beneficial and sustainable change to our health and well-being.

When you are balanced, you feel it. It is the absence of discordant sensations and emotions and the presence of a harmonious and calm unity. It is a feeling that brings relief and comfort.

The big blockage

As a physical and energetic process Qi Gong practice must start with work on the body to refine its natural mobility and functionality. The movements of much moderately dynamic Qi Gong, which is a good place to begin the study and practice, set out at first both to cultivate a deep level of relaxation (Fang Song) and restore good mobility, balance and co-ordinated movement. It often seems paradoxical that you are expected to practise specific and sometimes taxing movements while at the same time cultivating relaxation. It is an important early lesson in balancing the Yin of internal relaxing and the Yang of 'external effort' and movement. It is important that this relationship is considered in practice, since an excessive (and therefore Yang) use of muscle strength makes the business of learning the internal aspect (soft stretching flexibility and therefore Yin) difficult, if not impossible. Indeed it is the latter which is most important in Qi Gong. Giving up the normal reliance upon muscle strength and habitual tension, though, can be one of the most difficult hurdles.

Slow, rhythmic and mindful practice provides an ideal way of releasing long-term as well as daily tensions, but unless this is accompanied by proper release or a dissolving process the Qi Gong state will not be achieved. These tensions are mostly habitual but some tensions may be deep and old, resulting from accident, illness or emotional turmoil or shock, or they may be just the result of a stressful day. The slow movements of contracting and stretching, compressing and lengthening, loading and releasing, pushing and pulling, gently exercise the musculo-skeletal system, restoring tone and the lengthening capacity of the muscles, tendons, ligaments and connective tissue, as well as strengthening and increasing joint mobility and bone density.

Respiratory technique and harmonising of breath with movement plays an important role in refining the value of the movements and cultivates better oxygenation and gaseous exchange, with consequent benefits to our metabolism. Good respiratory technique also provides a tonifying and purgative massage of internal organs. This promotes good functionality and especially good digestion and elimination of waste. That same respiratory action promotes a healthy energetic, liquid tidal action throughout our bodies that not only supports the action of the heart but generally promotes the functional efficiency of all aspects of our system. Combined with gentle twisting and extending and contracting movements, Qi Gong stimulates and enhances endocrine secretion, lymphatic drainage and metabolic function in general, and consequently the homeostatic ability of the body.

Finally, by inhibiting mental activity (through cultivating a quiescent mental state) and using repetitive rhythmic movements enhanced by respiratory integration, Qi Gong restores the self-healing mode of the body, re-programming us to inhibit the common and (if engaged for too long) damaging stress mode which is now the cause of so much modern illness. Daily practice brings about restoration through the activities of the body's innate healing mode, which is our most precious and underused resource. Qi Gong teaches us to work on ourselves to increase our own capacity for self-healing and promote a healthy and optimally functional internal landscape.

> Qi Gong teaches energetic conservation and the distribution of our energetic resources to proiritize conservation, repair and replenishment. This can become a way of life and can both improve and change our daily life and how we deal with conflict and physical stress.

As a discipline, Qi Gong requires the allocation of dedicated time and a congenial location. In a busy day, finding the time to practise is difficult, but remember that a little bit often is better than a lot occasionally. Besides, after a while, just walking can become a Qi Gong and quiet moments can be used to 'go inside', to rest, recuperate, regenerate and switch off all the 'lights' for a while.

To achieve a high level of Qi Gong there is one last major obstacle to overcome. It is the most insidious of all obstacles in the achievement of Qi Gong. It is our own habitual preconceptions and internal dialogue that comprise much of our everyday mental activity.

As soon as you begin to regulate mental activity in accordance with Qi Gong practice it becomes very noticeable that the 'mind' is mischievous. Its undisciplined and self-gratifying and free-wheeling nature constantly conspires against anything that will expose its true nature. Mental activity in the form of an 'internal dialogue or commentary' typically wanders off in a distracted way, to duck and dive through the experiences and events that comprise our week, our day, our memories, projections and experiences. This often happens without us noticing a shift from a focused, mindful state to a dispersed and wandering mind state, when we discover that our mental activity has totally sabotaged our original intention. Cultivating the right Qi Gong mindset presents the biggest problem.

In dynamic Qi Gong it is easy to perform sets of movement without related mental activity. You could do a whole set of movements, for instance, and be thinking about anything but the movement. Similarly, in meditational or more quiescent Qi Gong it is easy to daydream and to become distracted. Until the mind is harnessed to the activity the Qi Gong will never be successful and will remain merely an exercise. Until the internal dialogue is quietened and the mental awareness is fine-tuned and focused, Qi Gong cannot be achieved and will remain superficial at best.

Relaxed, clear, aware and directing intelligence is critical to the success of Qi Gong practice. The depth of the Qi Gong experience is directly related to cultivation of a steady and uninterrupted mental focus.

Why bother to 'regulate' mental activity and inhibit or reprogramme our habitual mental activity at all? Beyond the health and mental well-being generated by Qi Gong, it softens the impact of the daily grind. Our experience of life often seems to 'happen' to us, and we often feel disconnected or somehow 'out of synch' with it. In extreme cases this can lead to depression and worse. We often feel overwhelmed by emotions and anxious, ungrounded and stressed. Bounced like a ping-pong ball between attraction and repulsion, we lose our clear judgement and ability to listen to what is really good for us and what we really need.

By inhibiting the runaway and mischievous 'monkey' nature of the mind through Qi Gong practice, we are able not only to conserve Energy but also to sense our true nature, relieved of the emotional and mental 'baggage' that we all end up carrying around.

Cultivating a sense of being 'rooted' or 'centred' and dissolving the negative residues of our years of living, refining and harmonising our functional and mental activity offers us a great sense of rejuvenation and internal strength and confidence. It is a process that not only enhances good health and happiness but also allows us to discover ourselves and recover the 'here and now' as a complete and fulfilling experience, undiluted and without distraction.

Reflect for a moment on the last time you really paid attention to what you were doing or the events unfolding moment by moment around you, fully aware and conscious of what you were doing as you were doing it, fully immersed, totally there with an attentive, intelligent awareness. This is not the same as being fully immersed emotionally, as in sudden anger, passion, sadness or an obsession, etc., where reflective awareness, a balanced engagement with the present condition and internal awareness are overwhelmed by a runaway, reactive emotional overload.

If you try and tell yourself moment by moment what you are doing, very soon you will be distracted and become absorbed in another train of thought. If you try and bring all your intelligent awareness to a single point of focus, either located within you physically or projected by your imagination, you will quickly realise how short is the time that you can honestly say you remained undistracted.

Inhabiting the moment means to be fully present in a psycho-somatic way, with all our energetic potential focused and alert, not squandered or dispersed irresponsibly. It is hard both to be here now, and to be now here. Bringing the emotional and distracted mind under control is a very difficult task.

Quiescent awareness is the initial meditational method employed to cultivate the correct mind for Qi Gong practice. It is a point of balance that is simultaneously a resting state and a state where all our energetic potential is available. Without the ability to cultivate the quiescent state, shut down the external noise and dissolve internal dialogue, there can be no real and deep Qi Gong.

We are encouraged from our early years to look outwards and to generally ignore our 'inner workings', for we learn very early on that they generally look after themselves. All we have to do, so to speak, is to drive the 'car'. We can live life without really being conscious of it.

The Qi Gong community believes that endlessly looking out depletes our life Energy and, via our senses, emotions and lifestyle, disperses our precious vital Energy – rather like water out of a bucket with holes.

The business of developing this quiescent state and subduing the 'inner dialogue' is without doubt the most difficult challenge of Qi Gong practice. It must be encouraged from the beginning, since it enables us to cultivate our vital Energy, activate our self-healing ability and direct our Energy for either martial, medical or Spiritual purposes. High-level practitioners are able to slip easily into this mind-frame, and indeed feel as if it is always present as a background, still and calm, regardless of what other distractions or events impinge upon them.

The biggest block to progress is our inability to look inwards and maintain a steady awareness to the exclusion of all else. It is the single most difficult aspect of practice, and the most vital, for it is the resulting quiescent state that will determine the success or failure and depth of our Qi Gong practice.

For beginners the easiest Qi Gong forms are the mildly dynamic sets with fixed feet positions, because the circular and spiralling movements both give a deep pleasure and also afford health benefits if practised properly. The movements fulfil our deep need to feel our physical self, mobile and functionally co-ordinated. Cultivating awareness of movement and internal sensations is the beginning of regulating the body, breath and mental activity.

Dynamic Qi Gong is very valuable since it builds muscle tone and develops flexibility, co-ordinated movement and integration of breath and function. But to really get to grips with it and nourish the vital Essence and Energy, we need to engage our intelligence and direct our awareness internally, to feel what is happening when we move in certain ways and to refine our movements in accordance with the subtle energetic sensations that arise from different types of movement. There should be no external distraction, lest our attention, and thus our Energy, become dispersed. Qi Gong to music, for instance, does not promote the right mental activity but creates just as much distraction as a plane flying overhead. The effectiveness of Qi Gong cannot be attained by means of an external prop.

All Qi Gong begins with the technique of deep physical relaxation, either in motion or in stillness. This is difficult enough, but it is the prerequisite for the smooth and balanced distribution of energetic resources throughout the body. It is the primary condition for Energy cultivation and circulation. In addition, it is the background against which internal awareness can be developed and refined.

Different stages of practice and different types of Qi Gong bring different rewards, and the longer you practise, the more you begin to refine your physical movement, your breath and your mental state. All three move inexorably towards full integration when a more subtle awareness of the physical and energetic self emerges. Getting on the path and staying with it are the most important factors. A simple, dynamic Qi Gong set is an important first step on the Qi Gong path. The simpler the better. If you are too ambitious in the first instance, your progress will not match your expectations and you will become despondent. It is not unusual in China to see someone practise the same few movements over and over again, day after day, until they have both reaped the benefits and felt the value of those few movements.

Beyond learning a dynamic set of Qi Gong movements to facilitate the deep relaxation and co-ordination of breath and movement, the practitioner needs to build awareness of the energetic body through the refinement of physical movement. This is all about subtle sensations and not the gross sense of contraction and internal stress that accompanies overly dynamic physical movement. It is about sensing the subtle internal currents that are set in motion throughout the internal landscape by the slightest movement. This is a distinctive phase in the study of Qi Gong and must be achieved in order to be able to cultivate the guiding and inducing (Dao Yin) ability that advanced Qi Gong requires. This means harnessing the mental Energy to harmonise intention or idea with respiration and physical activity. It is the path to achieving the 'regulation' of body, breath and mind. In health terms this level of Qi Gong brings a sense of physical and mental well-being and an increased capacity for prolonged mental focus, as well as the ability to direct the flow of energetic currents and facilitate their influence upon the internal climate. This is most easily achieved in a mildly dynamic Qi Gong where physical stress is minimised and the emphasis is on the mental process. If the body is stressed it becomes very difficult to practise this all-important method.

This method may begin with a stationary posture and focused attention on regulating the Lower, Middle or Upper Dan Tian. The Lower Dan Tian, however, typically stands as the first and most important part of the body to develop awareness of and cultivate a sense of energetic abundance. There are at least six other common points on the body where awareness and control must be cultivated as a precursor to training a healthy and abundant circulation and balanced distribution of Energy throughout the body. There are:

Middle Dan Tian, behind the sturnum; Lao Gong, approximately in the centre of the palms; Bai Hui, on the top of the head; Hui Yin, between the legs; Yong Quan, on the soles of the feet; and Upper Dan Tian, between the eyebrows and towards the centre of the head. Refer to a book on acupuncture for a precise guide.

The next phase is to build an awareness of the currents or threads of connection that are cultivated and reinforced by sensation and idea. By creating the idea of energetic currents and connective threads, sensations and changes within the body become evident. By practising this over a long period of time, connectivities and internal currents become felt experiences. There are many Qi Gongs that can achieve this, and there are many ways of practising it. The key is the gentle, focused projection of the idea and the principle of guiding and inducing Energy.

Achieving this ability is important in the process of creating abundant and unhindered mobility and distribution of our Energy. It is also used to target organs and sensed energetic blockages to heal and maintain optimum health. More mysteriously, though, it is also used to circulate Energy along specifc roots to 'purify' and 'cool' the spine and brain and mental processes. In addition it unites and blends the pre-birth and post-birth Energy and unites conscious-ness with the Dao. This practice is most commonly associated with Daoist Spiritual practice, but it has enormous benefits in medical Qi Gong for healing and rejuvenation. Of course both medical and Daoist ambitions are health, mental well-being and 'Eternal Spring', but the path is also relevant to Spiritual fulfilment.

Right effort, right shape, right forms and feelings

Most forms and Qi Gong practice require the body to take up some-times complex shapes or postures and co-ordinate changes from one shape to another, creating a continuous, fluid and rhythmic set of forms. Postural requirements and basic fixed and moving step postures are always learned first. For instance, some Taiji forms (Taiji is here considered as a Qi Gong) have over 70 of these postures, and as many movements connecting these postures together. This complexity accounts for why many people cannot learn or maintain the practice. Luckily, there are many simpler forms to choose from in the realms of Qi Gong. Since Taijiquan is both a boxing form and used as a Qi Gong for health, it is important to remember that its original length provides a comprehensive vocabulary of boxing movements. It needed to be long, but Qi Gong does not necessarily need such complexity in order to be beneficial.

Most moving or dynamic Qi Gong requires strict adherence to postural alignment. Since form and posture is where everyone must start, it can often be quite challenging, for, although we may never need to think about our co-ordinative skills, when asked to take up postures and follow rules and undertake complex movements we may often discover that we are not as well co-ordinated as we thought. In fact, we may need to seriously reconsider much about how we feel and see ourselves when we start trying to achieve proper moving and standing forms.

As a consequence, it can take some time before beginners master some of the basic vocabulary of posture and movement, and then string them together so that they appear seamlessly linked in a continuous, flowing sequence. Once the postures are reasonably correct, the refining process must begin. Perhaps this never ends. After so many years, I still regularly have little revelations about the shape and movement that I am practising.

Intelligent awareness continuously brings insight and refinement to shape and form. Refined shape and form continuously brings insight.

Shape must be learned externally first and then rediscovered within yourself. Your body and mind may well rebel against it at first. However, you must take possession of it and understand its external shape and resultant internal dynamic. A feeling of growing comfort in the shape is a good test of whether you are correct or not, though be warned that this may take a few sessions and much solo practice. Obviously a good teacher is important here, to make corrections and adjust you. When the external shape is correct the internal sensations become possible. When the awareness of the internal feeling of the shape integrates with the external shape, then we can say that the shape is somehow illuminated or informed by the internal feelings. Intention sets up the shape, and awareness explores the commensurate sensations and in turn adjusts the shape to alter and refine those sensations. Internal connections are made and habitually distorted movement or postural defects can be addressed.

As one practises more and more, the shapes become illuminated by the free, easy nature and cumulative physical experience of the movement. In addition the flow of Energy around the body and the relaxed integration of external and internal factors begins to show. A Qi Gong master can tell your level by observing these qualities. Postures that are arrived at merely by looking at the external form are always mannered and appear hollow and meaningless, since they focus on the external appearance only. Although sometimes these postures can look beautiful and impressive, they are generally without energetic substance.

Studying form, shape and postural requirements is the first level of training, and unfortunately many people stop here, satisfied with the external and physical aspects of a discipline that offers so much more. The forms alone are often very beautiful and rewarding to perform, and to many students of Qi Gong and Taijiquan in particular, this is enough. Unfortunately this is only the tip of the iceberg. If you have the patience, the tenacity and the courage to go deeper, there is much to discover that can radically change your life, health and well-being for the better.

Forms and feelings; feelings and forms

In China there are many hundreds, probably thousands, of Qi Gong forms. As far as traditional Qi Gong goes, most forms are derived from Buddhist and Daoist roots, the Daoist root being the oldest. The best known of the oldest forms mimic the characteristic movements of a variety of animals to promote the characteristics of health, vigour and 'Spirit' exhibited by that particular animal. Fighting skills have also been built around the martial characteristics of animals, and this in itself goes some way to define Chinese martial arts and also explains their incredible variety and richness. Animals are constantly referred to, and movements in Qi Gong forms aim to emulate both mythical and real animals. Anyone who has practised any of the more dynamic moving Qi Gongs, like Taijiquan, will be aware that certain postures engender certain feelings that seem to be the result of making those postural shapes alone.

Making a shape can easily give us the sense of the animal, and perhaps connects us to a deeper atavistic memory. Almost as if there are archetypal shapes that promote certain physiological and mental states, some may be martial, some may be healing and some may be more Spiritual. Taking up a posture is more than a physical arrangement. It is attuning to a deeper and older memory of shape functionality and behavioural characteristics learned over millennia and bound into our innate mechanisms.

When animals move we are entranced by their grace and their total integration of intention and action. The cat is a favourite, and the nearest thing to a wild predator that most of us will see in daily life. Its smooth movements and casual athletic skill are a wonder to watch. In the hunt, as its gaze and adjusted posture indicate intention and potential attack, it is totally focused, while still aware of its surroundings and alert to changing conditions. Complete attentive stillness. It is beautiful to see. Pick up a cat that does not want to be handled and you are in for trouble. Like all animals, no matter how small, they can be difficult to restrain and dangerous. Of course they have evolved to survive and hunt and escape but the sum of their intention, responsiveness and their pliable, unified strength and in-stinctive response gives them remarkable power beyond their size. No wonder humans studied the characteristics and the energetic qualities of animals when they began to elevate their natural ability into healing, religious and martial endeavours.

In health practice also, the animal world seemed to hold many secrets. The tortoise moves slowly and its breath is imperceptible. It sleeps for long periods as if dead and then miraculously returns to life. Its lifespan exceeds our own. No wonder Daoists attributed to the tortoise extraordinary divinatory ability, exceptional health and longevity.

Qi Gong practitioners know that by adjusting our physical self, assuming a posture or making a particular movement we can affect our inner world – physiological, mental and energetic.

Mobility and co-ordination are the starting points for this work, and later for developing movement harmonised with breath and then with mental intention. In this way the foundation is laid for taking control of the damaging and dispersing effects of emotional and environmental stress, by balancing the way Energy is mobilised, circulated and apportioned throughout the body.

Qi Gong sets out to restore us and enable us to recover our innate self, to restore our totality and our natural ease within ourselves and within our environment, to restore our instinctive and natural ability, to promote and exercise our natural range of mobility, and to let us be as completely 'in' our action as is the animal that we observe and admire. We want to be aware, strong, in the present, in ourselves, healthy, healed and balanced within and without. It seems a lot to expect of ourselves, but this is the foundation of the ancient tradition of Qi Gong. The Daoists believed it was the knowledge of the 'ancients', and as such a profound cultural inheritance. Qi Gong aims to attain the natural state that we have all inherited, and from which we have strayed.

Systems of Qi Gong are generally designated as 'still' or 'dynamic' with many permutations in between. They can be further classified as belonging to the medical, Spiritual or one of the many martial schools. In the case of the martial schools Qi Gong is often described as 'external' or 'internal'. The difference lies with the method of cultivating a martially relevant Energy and the characteristics of martial power.

The external schools rely upon speed, muscle force and overt power. They cultivate this by practising forms in a vigorous and dynamic way. Beautiful to watch, you can see and feel their power, speed and agility. Externally oriented Qi Gong is used to promote co-ordination, stamina, physical power and resilience to hard blows. Internal Qi Gong, by contrast, begins with softness and relaxation designed to foster internal Energy or at least the awareness of it, primarily in the torso and specifically in the Dan Tian. It too cultivates martial power and speed, but as the end products of a long, slow process of body adjustments aimed first at the soft (Yin), and then at the hard (Yang). Balancing soft Energy (Rou) and hard Energy (Gan) is characteristic of the internal schools.

The power of the internal school is cultivated first in the torso and later spreads to the arms and legs. Forms are generally practised slowly to develop a natural, elastic strength that relies upon contact with an opponent and a distinct sense of internal connectivity to the ground, and mind control over body response and movement. It is no less beautiful to watch than the external forms, being typified by a soft, smooth and continuous circular fluidity of movement with great emphasis placed upon the ability to change shape, function and direction with ease. The only problem with watching internal boxing styles, especially Taiji at a high level, is that it is difficult to see how it can be martial, since external movement is optimised to the minimum. When it is shown martially it can be difficult to see what exactly is done to repel an opponent. Consequently, it can look mysterious.

Methods and levels

Generally speaking, most dynamic Qi Gong relies upon natural mobility and co-ordinative skills. This can mean moving only the upper body while standing in certain fixed positions, or legs and upper body moving together with stepping or adjusting the foot-work to facilitate full body rotation. Arms may be extended, opened, drawn in and closed or raised and lowered. Often one arm may be extended while the other is withdrawn, or raised while the other is lowered. These gestures are often accompanied by stepping forward or sitting back, with one leg at any one time carrying more weight than the other. Body alignment is important and we will discuss this in detail in the next chapter. Upper and lower body co-ordination is harmonised by the rotational function of the pelvis.

It should be noted that dynamic Qi Gong generally exploits the full range of joint mobility and stretching to bring about beneficial effects on the muscles, tendons, ligaments and connective tissue, and in turn on the organs and the nervous and liquid systems of the internal landscape. Much of the physical postural work is relatively simple, especially in medical Qi Gong, which relies upon simple and natural movement. Its primary function is to de-stress, mobilise Energy and blood and promote respiration and homeostasis. Martial Qi Gong has a more pressing agenda which often requires the development of a type of Energy (Jin) that has a direct value in attack and defence applications. Spiritual Qi Gong is closer to medical Qi Gong, and indeed, the cultivation and circulation of Energy, breath and mental focus is the first level, though meditation (a still Qi Gong) is required to take it further.

The key to success in Qi Gong is first, the importance of relaxation and second, repetition. Typically a set of movements should be performed in a relaxed way while still fulfiling the required shape, but its repetition over five, ten, fifty or even a hundred times allows the relevant muscle groups to engage, at the same time minimising the effort required to achieve the form. Obviously too many repetitions are counter-productive since they tire the muscles, and too few are not enough to re-programme the neurological connections. The slow repetition and conscious relaxation of the whole body, and specifically of those areas where muscles are engaged, allows the mind to reduce the stress and strain involved in movement. After a period of regular practice it requires less effort to achieve the same movement, and so the movement of an arm, for instance, finds its optimum rotation, so as to engage and stretch the muscles without tiring them. Once this level is achieved progress becomes more subtle and a more refined physical and energetic awareness can be developed.

In addition to working the body, the movements should be done in accordance with the breath. Generally speaking this means abdominal breathing, but reverse breathing is also preferred in some methods of Qi Gong. The characteristics of the breath should be that it is long, silent, soft, deep and even. Inhalation normally accompanies a drawing-in motion, for instance, pulling the hands towards the body, while exhalation is accompanied by an extending motion – simple rules which are sometimes difficult to apply with complex co-ordination, but through relaxed practice the body is most often able to bring movement and breath into harmony. Careful observation and awareness of the relationship between breath and physical movement is as important to the first levels of practice as to the higher levels, and to practise Qi Gong without breath awareness is to ignore the cultivation of the second of the Three Treasures, Vital Breath (Qi).

Practice must be accompanied by an intelligent awareness. Qi Gong forms should never become just a set of movements. The mind must be focused and attentive to the activity. Depending on the type of Qi Gong, it should be actively engaged either in both sensing and directing the internal activity of movement, or thinking it. By thinking the form it is possible not only to perfect its outer shape but also to create an internal sense of total body connectivity and internal movement. Breath is the functional link between thought and movement. As such it should feel as if it is reaching all parts of the body and, directed by mental intention, actively impact upon any point or thread where the mind is focused. In many forms of Qi Gong, especially medical, the mental focus is directed to different acupuncture points to create internal energetic connections (Dao Yin).

Finally, a word about Taijiquan as a Qi Gong. Taiji is probably the most complex Qi Gong there is in terms of shape, co-ordination, variety and duration. Like all forms it can be done either with careful attention or mindlessly, as a mere set of movements. Whether it is practised as a martial art or as a pure Qi Gong it must incorporate correct posture, correct and co-ordinated breathing and correct mental focus. Without these conditions it will never suffice as a subtle martial art or as an advanced-level Qi Gong.

Five essentials and more

What follows is adapted from Grand Master Ma Yueh Liang's Five Character Maxim (Ma and Zee 1990). (Ma Yueh Liang was a third generation Master of Wu Style Taijiquan and senior disciple of Wu Jian Quan, founder of the modern Wu Style.)

Persevere

If you want to catch the meaning of Taijiquan you must persevere. It does not come all at once but in bits, like a jigsaw puzzle. You often do not see the full picture until much later.

Studying in China meant going to meet my teacher in the park every day, just as the sun was rising, without fail. In the park I see the same faces in the same places doing their morning practice. Many of them recognise me and I them, as they have seen me come and go since the early 1990s. Their practice is both a social event and private time for themselves, a peaceful interlude before the city gets into full swing, and a chance to practise their Qi Gong and Taijiquan. Their aim is simply good health and 'Eternal Spring': to be healthy and fit, with a clear mind, for as long as their time on this Earth allows them. We would all wish for the same.

Their daily routine is relaxed and unhurried and only measured by the sense of well-being that their regular practice brings. Each day's practice is an end in itself and, like eating rice, it is a normal daily activity – unless of course it is really cold, wet or windy. They know the value of daily practice and know that without persevering in their practice, nothing can be achieved. In parks across China this early morning scene can be witnessed. Some of the people I see in the park are seriously ill or frail, but under the guidance of a Qi Gong instructor they are working at recovery, or at least sustaining themselves as best they can. Some people can relate tales of remarkable recovery from serious illness by a daily regimen of Qi Gong, and many people believe that by cultivating Qi and practising the three regulations of body, breath and mind, it is possible to impact upon terminal illness as well as the more common seasonal complaints – or indeed, just the aches and pains of old age. It is, as one might expect, mostly middle-aged or older people who are the regulars. Taiji and other forms of Qi Gong are not often pursued by the young, whose sight is trained much more on the new wealth of China. I expect that when they get older and realise that you cannot buy health and well-being, they might turn to their cultural heritage for a solution.

In China perseverance is greatly admired. It is a sign of sincerity, and that is more valuable than talent or any amount of words, since talent is ephemeral and words do not always tell the truth. Persistence, however, proclaims intention and integrity. Perseverance furthers one, and this is especially true in the world of Qi Gong. Perseverance is therefore the critical factor.

There will always be students who are incredibly enthusiastic to learn but who cannot sustain their enthusiasm when it comes to self-practice. There are those with natural talent for movement who seem to learn quickly and easily, taking on the role like an actor, but whose talent becomes an obstacle which they cannot surmount: they become stuck in their own perception of what they are and what they are doing. Then there are those who come with good intention but can never quite concentrate or try hard enough to achieve the first level: they become dependent on the class and each visit is like the first time, but what they learn they leave behind. They remember nothing. The best student is the student who comes with an open, intelligent mind and a willingnesss to give solid effort, not maximum effort, to see what happens when you take the first and then the second step, for they have the mindset to continue if their imagination is caught by the practice and they will be drawn along the path of learning, enjoying each moment with no need to keep an eye on a goal. In this way time passes, and eventually form is achieved, and then, without desperation, more and more. Realisation dawns slowly, and without perseverance there can be no rewards.

Be precise

Since the benefits of Qi Gong are cumulative, regular practice is important if you are to accrue those benefits. Repetitive practice is the way forward and is the only way to refine the forms once they have been learned. Learning a form, however, is only the first step. Practising it correctly over and over again brings the benefits and the insights which propel you further. However, perseverance in wrong practice can be disastrous and leave you wondering what it is all about. Therefore it is important that you find a teacher you can trust and who knows enough to teach the foundations thoroughly and accurately. It is said in China that to miss in the beginning by an inch could mean ending up out by a mile. It is also said that it is better to learn one form well and understand it than learn ten forms and know nothing. Very true. There is often an eagerness to learn as much as you can as quickly as possible, but meaning and insight will elude you if your goal is purely acquisition. A competitive and acquisitional stance may impress some people, but to the wise it will appear without substance. Knowledge, insight and skill come from experience and depth of practice.

$\mathcal{T}$he starting point for Qi Gong is always the body, the shape and the guiding principles of relaxation and alignment. Getting these right refines functionality and being precise ensures the results.

Correct shape is often practised first in static postures to allow time for you to acquaint yourself with the postural requirements and recognise how to optimise the stresses and strains of each posture. Precise adjustment of the body can significantly change the different sensations that each posture produces. Refining those sensations through first gross and then subtle physical adjustment is an important aspect of learning and continual refinement, and something that we should keep to as our practice matures.

Some postures may be difficult for some and easy for others. Everyone will find difficulty somewhere. Starting from fixed postures is a good way to put a group all at the same starting point. Precise posture, however, must also apply to transitional movement, and this is harder to achieve. Correct relationships to the central line and optimum curves and rotations are all difficult to achieve for the beginner. The shape of both static posture and posture in movement must be continually refined and observed.

In seeking precision it is easy to neglect legs and feet in favour of hands and arms, since we are very used to using our hands and typically pay less attention to our legs and feet, and especially to our pelvis, which provides the functional link between the two. Since a main first objective of Qi Gong is to harmonise upper and lower body, arms and legs, hands and feet, it is important to pay attention to how they link and function together, rather than in isolation.

Many students may at first feel that some of the shapes of Qi Gong, and the need to constantly monitor posture, are too difficult. It is certainly a lot to take on, and so it is always best to develop the overall body awareness slowly. In Taiji, for instance, one of the most difficult and demanding of all Qi Gongs, certain postures may feel uncomfortable and even unstable to the beginnner. Certainly many of the shapes or foms we assume are not easily found in our normal daytime activity. Nevertheless, the shapes of Qi Gong and Taiji are designed to impact upon our physiological, psychological and energetic state. In order for them to do this effectively we must get them right, and for that we must cultivate a total body awareness.

Taijiquan has the added agenda of being a martial art, so its postures and movements are all designed to comply with attack and defence.

Many people have the idea that Qi Gong, and especially Taijiquan, movements are somehow inexact, and that it is all just 'floating about' and waving your arms in a sort of physically liberating free movement. Nothing could be further from the truth. It is an exacting and demanding skill based upon strict rules and principles, and it may seem something of a paradox that the pursuit and application of those strict guiding principles re-educates the body to become more free and liberated. At a certain point, as in many creative disciplines, many of those rules that are so important in the early years can later be relaxed, since they will have by then become fully assimilated and natural to you.

Correct posture, optimised and integrated movement, is deeply satisfying, not least in that it brings us a new awareness of our physicality and a new pleasure in simply moving.

Be slow

To cultivate precise movement and posture, Qi Gong and Taiji are practised slowly. More specifically, movement is harnessed and driven by the rhythms of your inhalation and exhalation.

Slow practice allows time to monitor posture and refine movement. It is this characteristic of slow movement that most people identify with Qi Gong, and especially Taijiquan, and which has given rise to the idea that Taijiquan could not possibly be a martial art. Slowness is a strategic method of practice, since it allows time for accuracy of movement and refining the sense of balance, as well as being an effective way of stimulating the metabolism and the self-healing mechanism of the body.

The slow exchange of weight from one leg to the other in moving Qi Gong, and the deliberate rotational extending and withdrawing or convergence and divergence of the arms, combined with turning of the torso, gently warms and retrains the body to minimise exertion. Slowness allows time to consciously relax the body and harmonise the movement to the breath and mental awareness and intention. As form practice is prolonged, the breath noticeably slows, and consequently so does movement.

Slowness allows the discernment of weight distribution and of how we are balanced at any one moment within our movement. It allows us time to be aware, without the accompanying physical exertion of more stressful exercise, of the stretching and contracting, pulling and pushing, opening and closing sensations, and of the refinement of circular and rotational movement. These are all aspects of our normal physical mobility, but done in a way that allows us to minimise effort while increasing functionality.

Finally, slowness of movement increases load bearing and therefore strengthens the joints and bones, which is especially important as we get older. It builds elastic and flexible strength in the legs, as opposed to muscle bulk, and it promotes a softer torso musculature through the requirement of relaxation, which reverses our propensity, probably resulting from lifestyle, cultural preference and bad breathing habits, to carry excessive tension in the chest and to build too much muscle bulk there at the expense of the rest of the body. Slowness allows investigation of sensations and brings an awareness of areas of increased tension and energetic stagnation. This gives us the chance to begin the business of dissolving deep tensions as well as easing postural difficulty.

Be light

Novice students and passing critics of Taijiquan are often surprised at the level of strength and stamina needed to practise Taijiquan forms accurately and slowly, when they try it for themselves. In fact they are using excessive strength and their movements are not integrated, so they feel the accompanying compensatory tension and strain, whereas a regular and mature practitioner will have little trouble in completing a form and should feel energised afterwards. In addition, the experienced practitioner will feel light, though not a floating sort of lightness: the lightness will be felt throughout the body, but the feet will feel firmly in touch with the ground (though not as if stuck in mud).

Lightness is in fact a characteristic of Qi Gong, both as a sensation felt within the practitioner and as a quality that is evident to a viewer. Lightness is developed through practice and is the result of correct body alignment and structure, relaxation, rounded and curved movement and an appropriate mental state.

Lightness is as much a state of mind as it is a sensation of the body.

Lightness can also mean looseness – not the looseness of excessive mobility, but rather movement without stiffness. Qi Gong forms allow investigation into areas of stiffness, which is seen as stagnant or blocked Energy, so that internal mobility is felt as loose, free and responsive, without hindrance. Lightness is a physical sensation characterised by ease of movement and change, agility and an alert, intelligent mobility. The top of the head is key to achieving this, and lifting the acupuncture point known as '100 meeting places' (Bai Hui) at the very top of the head, as if it is suspended from above, gives a strong feeling of lightness and buoyancy in the legs. When lightness is achieved, agility can be nurtured. This is important for the martially oriented Taijiquan practitioner, for without agility the attack and defence methods and strategies will remain clumsy and unworkable.

In both practice and in daily life we should acknowledge this feeling. By holding the idea and 'suspending the top of the head' we can encourage the physical sensation. To feel light while still feeling connected to the ground is a very comfortable feeling and one that we can all appreciate, especially as we get older.

Be still

Ultimately, without stillness, perseverence, precision, lightness and slowness will not bear fruit. Stillness is the mother of movement and is the mind undistracted.

At the start of any Qi Gong practice the mind must be emptied of 'chatter' and distraction. The attention must be focused inward. This preliminary state reflects the original and undifferentiated state of emptiness (Wu Ji) before Taiji arises. The thought to move sees the separation of Yin and Yang and the emergent changing state that constantly separates but seeks balance and unity. By keeping a relaxed and still centre, balance and unity in movement can be achieved. In Taijiquan this is referred to as central equilbrium (Zhong Ding) and exists in every moment and movement. To retain it there must be 'aware stillness' and the movements must be restrained but complete. In Qi Gong terms this means no 'excess' and no 'deficiency' and 'everything arrives together' and 'everything starts together'. This simple rule ensures that the still centre is not compromised.

Feelings of imbalance generally indicate excessive muscle usage and consequent rigidity. They also show up poor co-ordination and integration of movement and, importantly, mean there is no sense of mental, and consequently physical, stillness. Generally the mature practitioner understands this and does the minumum externally to achieve the most internally. In this way the internal state has priority and stillness can be nurtured in relationship to movement. The beginner does too much externally and achieves very little internally.

*W*ithin the practice of Qi Gong and Taijiquan the idea of stillness is a critical requirement. It is a felt sensation and is the point from which a clear thought can mobilise movement to an exact measure, no more and no less.

It is the mental calm that settles the breath, it is the state of relaxation that dissolves tension, and it is the still, quiescent mind that stimulates healing and the free and natural circulation of Energy. When stillness presides, it is evident in movement. It is the fulcrum of perfect balance, whereby all disparate entities and convergent forces are reconciled.

In the beginning stillness is hard to achieve, since the work of focusing on the movement of the body, postural correctness, co-ordination and relaxation seem to challenge our habitual physical sense of ourself. Slowly, though, and as you become comfortable and familiar with the postures and transitions and they become hard-wired, then the mind can be trained, first by focusing on the Lower Dan Tian until the still centre of movement and the quiescent mind emerge and grow simultaneously. Once this foundation is laid, the mental focus becomes a guiding principle in both gross and subtle movement and also in guiding and inducing (Dao Yin) energetic change and balance to promote the conservation and optimum circulation of Energy. This is not an intellectual state in the conventional sense, where an idea is articulated in words, but more a sensed, nonverbal directing awareness that is a total body experience. At the centre of it all is a quiescent and still state that transcends the conventional dichotomy of mind and body.

These five points were originally expounded by Master Ma Yueh Liang and are embedded in the the methods of practice expounded by the Shanghai School of Traditional Wu Style Boxing. Although they refer to Taijiquan practice specifically, they also provide basic guidelines for all Qi Gong practice. For Qi Gong and Taiji to be really beneficial these five points must be observed and practised diligently, for they are the ground rules necessary for genuine practice. They are both literal and subtle in their meaning and must be studied to really make sense. They are all linked and support each other, for without any one the others would have less value.

More key principles for practice
USE THE MIND, NOT FORCE...

In stillness, the clear, unconfused mind is able to initiate movement correctly. In the beginning, the mind directs and creates the shapes, observes and feels them and mobilises and guides the changes from one posture to the next. The idea of movement and change must be held in a calm and coherent state. The body may appear to stop externally at the completion of a movement, but the mental intention is the transitional link to the next movement. In this way movements can be connected as if threaded together. When the body is trained to be relaxed, physically articulate, responsive to the subtle directing will (Yi), you have achieved the state of using the mind, not force.

Always, in Qi Gong and Taiji boxing (internal schools), the aim is to reduce the amount of strength, and consequently of effort used. Bringing the body into a natural state of trained comfort necessitates being aware of excessive use of strength (Li). There is an optimum level of exertion. Indeed, inadequate strength is as much of an error as excessive strength. Generally though, we are more prone to use excess strength in both our posture and our habitual action. In practice it is therefore important to avoid overexertion, since this trains muscular strength only and cultivates a coarse and unsustainable energetic quality. The saying 'Use the mind, not strength' effectively means: be as relaxed as you can while maintaining proper shape and structure, and direct the movements by using your mental intention (Yi Nian).

Qi Gong and Taijiquan are both physical and intellectual puzzles. For instance, how can you take up a position that is physically and co-ordinatively demanding while relaxing at the same time? It seems a contradiction. In time, however, it becomes apparent that we all overestimate the strength and tensions required, and when we give up our strength and let the mind more actively inform and infuse our posture, then we become more comfortable, and quickly we feel natural and at ease in what before felt awkward and unnatural. As you mature in practice, the relaxation and correctness of shape in posture and movement will allow you to perceive internal movement of Energy. Small, incremental adjustments to shape and levels of deep relaxation (Fang Song) will increase those sensations, leading to a greater and deeper internal perception and also a greater harmony between the internal sensations and the external movement. Eventually you establish connections within the body that give it the external characteristics of unified and fully integrated movement while, internally, Energy can be cultivated and balanced. In addition the physical and energetic properties can be applied to different ends, e.g. martial, healing or Spiritual cultivation.

For example, internal school martial arts, e.g. Taijiquan, Ba Gua or Xing Yi, are typified by their ability to change shape, function and direction seamlessly in attack or defence without loss of power or postural compromise. This requires the body to be supremely relaxed and soft in response to an opponent, and the ability to translate mental intention into action immediately, free of heavy muscular force and a ponderous thought process. Generally speaking the internal schools (Nei Jia) attach higher value to developing mental skill than to rigid martial applications, speed and muscular power. More on this later.

In Qi Gong practice, movement is led by the mental intention. Indeed, Qi Gong awareness is the blending of both the sense of and the thinking of the initiating and directing movement. In this way it is both sensed and thought. In traditional terms this relates to both the emotional, sensorily oriented mind and the intentful, volitional and higher mind, or fire and water, generally referred to as Xin and Yi (a faculty of Shen). All Qi Gong requires the emotional 'fire' aspect to be balanced and cooled by the intelligent, volitional wisdom mind, associated with water. This cannot be achieved by cultivating the coarse Energy of purely physical strength and excessively wilful effort. It is a long, slow process.

It is said that Qi Energy and blood go where the thought goes, and that without proper mental intention, Energy will disperse, inducing imbalance. Correct and focused intention has value both in self-healing and martial arts, as well as in Spiritual cultivation. It is at the very core of Qi Gong principles. For to succeed, the body and the mind must undergo balancing and regulating through correct training and practice. To achieve this is liberating and opens the door to a more powerful and meaningful practice.

Note

Traditional Chinese thinking does not separate the mind from the body in the way that traditional Western thinking does. Mental and sensory awareness, emotions, will, volition and intellectual ability are really embodied in the concepts of Xin and Shen (though some traditions identify Shen as pure Spirit only). This whole idea implies that thought is rooted in sensory and physical awareness. In addition, health and well-being are thought to be determined by the heart, which is both the governing organ of the body and a profound energetic centre and generator of physical, mental and energetic coherence – a state of total body intelligence. This clearly expresses a holistic view. Shen, however, is considered as Spirit, being a fundamental, pure state inherent in all of us, as well as a higher state of wisdom mind. Mental intention, so important in the practice of Qi Gong, is often referred to as Yi, which is generally associated more with the wisdom mind, Shen, than the more emotional heart–mind, Xin. Yi is the means both of taking control of the more emotional heart–mind, and of governing the physical, emotional and energetic body. It is also the bridge and the mechanism for informing the higher levels of consciousness (Shen).

POSTURE

After years of teaching and observing posture (and the accompanying mindset) it is natural now to notice the postural difficulties many people suffer from: the habitual tilt of the head, the rolling gait, the compensatory position assumed as the result of an injury, or of years of sitting badly at a computer, or just of years of sitting, etc. I look at how people stand, sit and breathe. Their physical presence registers as degrees of harmony and integration or disharmony and imbalance, and I am amazed at the discomfort that many people, especially (though not exclusively) older people, must feel. Sadly, it is also becoming more evident in young people who should be enjoying the natural mobility and vitality of their youth.

Through the practice of Taijiquan and Qi Gong you become aware of your own posture, breath and movement, and you naturally become curious about others.

Many people just do not look comfortable with their physicality. Most of us have experienced this at some point, generally as the result of an accident or illness or emotional turmoil that has left us emotionally scarred and somehow dislocated from our physical self. We are all subject to such eventualities. Sometimes they go away and sometimes they leave an imprint, held tight in the muscles and connective tissue of our body. The energetic and emotional content of injury or events can be retained. This psychosomatic memory can be debilitating. For instance, a fall that causes a back injury that constantly re-occurs when we move in certain ways will not only keep us continually on guard and restrict our range of movements, but we will lose confidence in our own functionality and physical ability. We may withdraw from activities we would normally get involved in, and walk in a way that compensates for the discomfort and perhaps pain that the event caused. Emotional trauma can have a similar effect, though perhaps more insidious. The imprint can remain long after we have forgotten the incident. I suppose we all carry the cumulative tensions of our life within us, not just locked in our minds, but as restrictive tensions locked into our very tissues.

We learn to live with them, and generally we can. However, as we get older we become more aware of deep tensions, and as we lose mobility those tensions seem to show through. We would undoubtedly all be more comfortable without the extra tensions that life leaves within us.

Qi Gong brings us into a state of awareness of our body and specifically our posture. The movements that comprise much Qi Gong are designed to release long-term and daily tensions, and the quiescent mind that is cultivated can assist in their dispersal and redress postural imbalances. In teaching, I have found that the release of old tensions can be both dramatic and emotional; or it can happen as a slow dispersal or dissolving with no evident emotional content. Generally all students find there is some sense of emotional release as the body recovers a looser, more relaxed state and the mind is able to focus on the internal landscape. The aim of practice is to disperse all tensions and to release muscle and other tissue from the restriction of spasm and trauma, whether physical or emotional, and regain a postural alignment and gait that will maintain an optimum state of health and promote the free and unhindered circulation of Energy. A lot of Qi Gong does this by engaging the whole body in continuous, rhythmic movement that crucially harmonises breath, movement and guided mental awareness so as to release through the whole body tissue matrix, rather than working on muscle groups in isolation.

Up until now in the West, there has been a poor health culture. We are more likely to be encouraged to run to a doctor for a consultation and take a drug. Non-involvement in our own health has led to a carefree view with a reliance on interventory and drug-based medicine and, also important, is the removal of personal involvement and responsibility from the equation.

Self-healing is a natural function of our body, at least within certain constraints, and we should be aware of it, cultivate and use it to promote our well-being. Qi Gong is the most accessible method, since it does not necessitate gymnastic skills or physical strength.

The complex patterns of movement and co-ordination that are required of Qi Gong and especially Taijiquan, owing to its complex physical vocabulary, make us very aware of our own physical ability. Studying Qi Gong prioritises our mobility, movement and co-ordination skills. Movement is our functional relationship with the world we live in, and it is through mobility that we experience much of our environment and what comprises our physical experience. Lack of mobility greatly reduces our ability to engage with the world and others. Taijiquan and Qi Gong put emphasis on recovering and building upon our natural co-ordination and normal range of mobility. Practice is like peeling off layers of restrictive habitual tensions in our body and revealing the simple co-ordinative and movement skills that most of us are born with and develop comfortably as we grow, unless or until we lose touch with ourselves. Such co-ordinated mobility is deeply satisfying and pleasurable.

Internally, Qi Gong promotes mobility in the liquid and tissue world of our interior landscape: blood, fluids, muscle, tissue, organs and cells, all moving in rhythms of the mutual harmony that is the pulse of our life. It is possible not only to sense whether there is internal harmony or disharmony, but to affect it beneficially through the methods of Qi Gong.

Qi Gong and Taijiquan develop harmonious and integrated movement and increase our flexibility and mobility to correct postural anomalies and release spontaneously the residue of injury, emotional trauma and general stress held within us.

In our modern Western world, physical activity has been minimised by mechanisation and it has become hard to maintain an overall balanced relationship of muscles. Muscle tone and ability are preserved only if demands are placed upon them by our activity or the environment. Natural relationships of muscles suffer and imbalance becomes a normal sense of our physical selves. Excess muscle tension is common, as is undue stress on the joints and bones. Taiji and Qi Gong not only promote body awareness but give us the means to affect the body holistically.

The postural requirements of Qi Gong are considered fundamental to inner cultivation and the nourishment of vital Energy, for they are the first requirements of body work and must become habitual and natural in all forms and movement. Since the practice of Qi Gong is also about our daily lives and well-being we must translate the lessons of practice into our ordinary lives.

Simply standing up

According to traditional Daoist thinking we are a microcosm of the universe, and therefore subject to the influences and Energy of the 'Heavens' as much as the Earth. We absorb from above and from below and are influenced accordingly. Both are considered a source of Energy, and within us the reconciliation and balanced use of those energies is assumed as a natural part of living. Indeed, these energies are referred to as Qi and are as important to our well-being as food and water. Our bioelectrical, biochemical and biomechanical selves are profoundly influenced by our environment, both that above us and that below us. The principles of proper postural alignment are designed specifically to optimise the physical and energetic systems of the body. The more open and receptive the body to beneficial elements from the environment, the more readily we can nourish our own Energy through the methods of self-cultivation.

Simply standing is considered the fundamental posture of Qi Gong. It makes sense, since that is what we do much of the time. Whether in stillness or in movement, standing up or, let us say, staying upright, is important to our ability to optimise the stress and strain of our mass against the pull of gravity and to maintain that in motion. Our ability to stand up has formed our physiology, our culture and the environment. In Qi Gong, there are important guidelines for creating the perfect standing posture, which not only facilitates the efficient dispersal of our mass downwards, but also optimises, in the opposite direction, the ability to stay upright that defines our species.

In addition these fundamental postural conditions have both mechanical and energetic value, in that correct postural conditions permit the free and natural generation and movement of Energy throughout our internal systems. The following are the basic postural conditions for achieving this.

Suspend the head

'Suspending the head' is considered one of the main postural requirements in Qi Gong. It means that the physical sensation of ourselves, when the head is correctly positioned, is that of being pulled up or suspended by a thread from the sky so that, as in a string puppet, everything hangs from that point. More accurately, our skeleton feels as if it is uplifted, while our skeletal muscles should have a sinking downward sensation. The main feeling, however, is in the spine, which should feel lengthened by the complementary feelings of being pulled up from the cervical vertebrae while sinking downwards from the lumbar region and sacrum. It is as if the spine is being stretched from both ends. The point on the top of the head known poetically as '100 meeting places' (Bai Hui), sometimes called the Head Star, is the highest point on a line drawn over the head from the top of one ear to the other. It is an important point, both in acupuncture and as the balancing axial top point by which we can understand our verticality, position and mobility in space. At the beginning, when studying Qi Gong and Taijiquan it is not advisable to focus incessantly on one point until the external forms are cultivated. However, as you proceed there are various points on the body that become self-evidently important. Bai Hui is one of those points, and you will find that in both standing and dynamic Qi Gong and Taijiquan, a developed awareness of this point is critical to cultivating Energy and mobilising it, as well as developing form precision, lightness and agility in movement.

The correct feeling cannot be achieved if, for example, you pull the chin in too far or to tensely, or if your chin protrudes. The neck should feel comfortable and, if anything, 'empty'. This is the feeling of the weight of the skull and its contents being dissolved down through the spine efficiently and optimally. I mention this because beginners, when asked to pull up the point Bai Hui, often stick out their chin to tilt the head backwards. The head can be put into position by a teacher to acclimatise the student. However, lifting or suspending the head alone cannot bring about the right internal sensation unless the second postural requirement is in place.

Inside sinking

Imagine a plumb-line from the point Bai Hui through your body. The top of the line is somewhere far above you and the line passes out of your body at another important point called Hui Yin ('Yin returning') between your legs (located between your genitals and anus). Now imagine a plumb-line suspended from the sky. When the two points Bai Hui and Hui Yin are in line, then we are properly aligned vertically, and we will know this because the progressive relaxation of the skeletal muscles that keep us erect will allow the weight of our torso, head and arms to be comfortably dissolved downwards into the ground. Our feet and legs will take up the weight as our upper bodies begin to feel lighter. The feet may feel as if they are half sunk in or stuck to the ground, and this is called our 'root'. It is the point where our downward weight meets the supporting quality of the Earth.

The rising and sinking sensation felt in the body that results from lifting or suspending the head, accompanied by the complementary feeling of sinking downwards, provides a sense of elongation, the fulcrum of which is our centre point, known as Lower Dan Tian or Elixir Field. It is probably the single most important area to cultivate and be aware of in beginner and intermediate Qi Gong.

There is a distinct sensation of this centre which grows as one's practice matures. I will come back to the Lower Dan Tian in the next chapter, but for now it is enough to know that 'sinking Qi to Dan Tian' means to contact this point of sensation, when the body feels clearly suspended from Bai Hui, with an accompanying sensation of downward sinking brought about by relaxing the muscles, especially the abdomen and the diaphragm. Sinking Qi to Lower Dan Tian also requires abdominal breathing (see the section 'Simply beathing' on pages 127–132) and an accompanying feeling that you are inhaling all the way into the Lower Dan Tian area. Of course this is not possible, since the lungs do not extend this far, but the sensation of deep, abdominal breathing serves, along with firming the vertical axial thread and the sensation of Lower Dan Tian as an energetic center, to bring about the feeling of Energy in the torso sinking into the lower abdomen and down to the feet.

Note

Both these first two principles are relatively easy for a sincere and sensitive practitioner to catch at an early stage. As the practice matures and becomes more refined, the sensations deepen. In addition, how suspending the head and cultivating that internal sinking sensation informs your Qi Gong and Taijiquan becomes more and more clear and formative as you develop the correct structuring of the body in movement and stillness. It is common for beginners to be careless about these two criteria, but they are fundamental to the methods of inner cultivation (Nei Gong).

Relax the shoulders

This means to allow your shoulders to sink downwards and to hang naturally. One of the first and most habitual signs of stress in the body is the raising and tensing of the shoulders. This is so normal in most people that they are no longer aware of it. In many cases, even when you believe your shoulders are hanging naturally, they are not. Tension in the shoulders not only denies the practitioner the connective inner thread from Bai Hui to Hui Yin and the sense of Lower Dan Tian, but it also reduces the energetic connection and exchange between the head and the body and the arms and the torso. Habitual tension in the shoulders can cause headaches, a serious sense of discomfort, distortion of posture and restricted respiration.

In all instances and most especially in Qi Gong (as well as Taiji boxing practice), relaxed shoulders are a must. Even when the arm is raised, the shoulder must be trained to remain relaxed and the joint to feel open and mobile. This is hard and is a relatively advanced ability, especially when the arm is raised above shoulder level. It is important that the natural tensions required to do this must not be supplemented by over-tensing the muscles. The area around the shoulder joint must be gently pulled 'open' and not restricted by excess tension.

I constantly remind students to relax their shoulders, since it is easy to forget. There are, however, degrees of relaxation, and even when one maintains awareness and can practise dropping the shoulders, it will take some time before that can be applied to all our daily activities – which is where the practice must end up if these principles are going to help nourish and conserve our life Energy and get us through the day with minimum tension.

Relax the chest

With the shoulders relaxed, the chest can also be relaxed, allowing a sensation of openness and comfort. Like shoulder tension, chest tension is very common indeed. Both are generally related, and both can serve to restrict adequate and efficient respiration, which is contradictory and counter-productive to the practice of Qi Gong. Typically in the West when we are instructed to stand upright, we thrust out our chest, raising the sternum, expanding the rib-cage and pulling the shoulders back. It is a kind of puffing up to make ourselves look bigger and more powerful. This is alien to the postural requirements of Qi Gong.

Generally speaking, the relaxed chest means the sternum is not raised and the rib-cage is relaxed. Combined with relaxed abdominal muscles and shoulders, breathing becomes easier and more efficient, with the diaphragm able to move unrestricted.

Pull up the back

This idea is a difficult one and should not be treated in isolation, indeed none of these postural requirements should be. They are all intimately connected and contingent on each other. In Qi Gong the back should be relatively straight while retaining its natural thoracic and lumbar curves. However, Qi Gong postures do require you to reduce excess curvature, while retaining the natural flexibility and mobility of the spine. It is a common mistake to artificially flatten the back when it is wholly contrary to the spine's natural condition. However, in most cases some adjustment to the back is to be recommended, though it must be done with proper care and attention and is best done over a long period of practice as the whole body adjusts and awareness is increasing. The best way to achieve this is by adjusting the pelvis.

'Pull up the back' really is a sensation that results from the cumulative effects of suspending the Bai Hui point, relaxing the shoulders, allowing the chest to relax and open comfortably, plus the general sinking sensation brought about by relaxation. It does not literally mean to lift up the back, but there is a sense that the area is slightly expanded and broadened out to link to the arms, and also the sensation that the back, especially the thorax, is functionally related to the chest. The sense of being wrapped by the ribs and the associated muscles, plus the consequent relaxing, opening and lengthening sensation of connectivity between the upper back and the sacrum, down the long bony spine and associated muscles, nerves and connective tissue, cultivates a strong sense of Energy, like the fulcral point in the upper back. It is a lifting sensation.

Straighten the tail-bone

We have all grown accustomed to, though not necessarily comfortable with, the way our lower spine is set, and so this recommendation is often hard to implement and hard to maintain. Generally speaking it entails rotating the pelvis under slightly, which in turn turns the coccyx (Wei Lu) downwards. It should not be done too emphatically, since this can cause discomfort and unnecessary tension. Critically, it should be comfortable and accompanied by as much relaxation in the upper body as you can achieve at your stage of development. This requirement is about angling the pelvis in such a way that it can function properly as a platform for the upper body, allowing the weight to be efficiently dissipated downwards throughout the structure.

Indeed, when the coccyx and consequently the pelvis are correctly angled, the sense of lightness in the upper body and the increased sense of support and compression in the legs is verification of the correct position. It is definitely a point of fine-tuning which becomes very important in cultivating a free and unhindered circulation of Energy, and also in locating and firming the area of Lower Dan Tian.

Over-emphatic turning under is as much of an error as leaving the pelvis protruding, either of which would denote an inefficient pelvic angle, unable to play a proper role in controlled mobility and the cultivation of loose strength. When Wei Lu is properly positioned, the body will feel relaxed. The upper body will feel light and lively, and the lower body loose, strong and mobile. Upper and lower body will feel connected, and the lower back will feel full.

Finally, the pelvis must stay at all times horizontal to the floor so that it can provide a stable platform and a constant level in pelvic rotation. It is a common error, in shifting weight to one side, for the pelvis to lose its horizontality and the hip-joint to become locked, with the hip-bone of the weighted side unnaturally lifted or pushed out. Keeping the pelvis correctly adjusted as a rotational platform in standing and movement is incredibly important in Qi Gong and Taiji boxing.

Do not lock the joints

In Qi Gong the joints are never locked back, since this would deny them mobility and constrict the muscles and tendons immediately surrounding the joints. The joints are considered as Energy gates through which Energy is transferred, and consequently any restriction will reduce or inhibit the flow of that Energy. Also, the principle of relaxed and rounded movement is best served by the arms and legs being slightly bent. This allows for functional expansion and lengthening and folding. In addition, from a martial point of view, locked joints are vulnerable to damage and breaking. They also restrict agility and spontaneous responsive movement.

A sinking sensation

Postural alignment must be taught from the beginning. It is key to all the postures, and as such is considered part of the 'external' or postural aspect of Taiji and Qi Gong. Correct posture, besides, opens the door to awareness of the resulting 'internal' sensations and ability to cultivate the 'right' sensations. The most important and first sensation that must be cultivated is a sense of 'internal sinking'. We have alluded to this in 'sink Qi to Dan Tian', but we need to look more closely at what it means and how to get to it.

The sense of 'sinking' (Song Jin) is the primary condition of all Qi Gong and Taijiquan, and it is the direct result of relaxing of the muscles downwards against the upward push of the skeleton. The most common instruction in Qi Gong and Taiji practice is probably Song, which is used to denote generally 'relax'. 'Relax' (Fang Song) results in sinking, and the more you can relax while keeping proper skeletal alignment, the more you cultivate the feeling of sinking. Sinking, incidentally, does not mean that the head drops and the body lowers, it means that the muscles relax their contraction to an optimum level, sufficient to maintain postural integrity and minimise 'stress and strain' in standing, moving and in the performance of lifting, pushing and pulling tasks. In other words, it is a state that is desirable for our daily existence and not just for the times we practise Qi Gong or a set of Taijiquan. Furthermore, the state of sinking is a state of alert relaxation, not the sleepy, restful state that we might normally associate with the term 'relax'. In sinking, the body is relaxed, centred and alert. The best analogy is that of a cat: soft, flexible, relaxed and apparently contemplative, yet fully aware of its surroundings.

To continue with the cat. When the cat walks along a narrow fence and you stroke it or apply any lateral pressure to it, you can feel it sink its centre to accomodate the force. If you increase the pressure it will lower its body in accordance with the increased pressure; it will retain its composure and its balance. It knows where its physical centre is at all times. The aim in Qi Gong and most especially Taiji boxing is to achieve something similar.

Being relaxed allows us to feel as if we are sinking downward and growing 'roots' into the Earth. It gives a sense of being fully grounded, which, surprisingly, makes you feel light in the upper body (whereas excess tension literally makes you feel as if you are being weighed down). Acquiring this state also strengthens the legs, rather like a spring, allowing the muscles to stay naturally long and not compacted in the way that certain types of training can. The practice of sinking brings the upper body into a precise functional relationship with the legs, whose springy strength is co-ordinated by the waist, to allow power from below to be transmitted to the upper body with minimum muscle effort required. The accompanying energetic sensation resulting from relaxed sinking is a strong sense of body integration and an accompanying sense of internal relief, since the organs are relieved of being held in unnatural tension and are able to function and move more comfortably.

The downward sinking and upward rising quality are best explained by the Yin–Yang theory, simultaneously felt as complementary but opposing forces. Downward sinking is made possible by upward pushing. If there is sinking there must be rising, if there is rising there must be sinking.

For an infant, learning to stand and walk is a new and acquired feeling that quickly gets forgotten in new stages of growth and achievement. To reconnect with that sensation is as thrilling in maturity as it must be for a child.

Sinking, then, is a very physical and basic physiological sensation. Sinking connects us to the ground, our feet feel 'rooted' deep into the Earth. When we walk our legs feel strong and springy and responsive to the downward force of gravity acting upon our mass, reconciled and balanced by our upwardly aligned verticality. We take all this for granted, but the realms of Qi Gong, and especially the complex moving forms like Taijiquan, make us very aware of our own sense of balance (Zhong Ding) in space. We have to re-think and re-experience how it feels to be stable and upright. When fully matured through practice, the sensation is strong. We feel our architecture and our 'tone' – the internal structures and tensions that hold us in shape.

When we lift our arms up high, there may be an accompanying sense of lightness generated in the legs, as if the whole of our body is following the rising arms. Our chest and shoulders will feel the strain, and muscle groups will work together to get the arms up as efficiently as possible. Consequently we may feel slightly disconnected from the ground, as if Energy is all rising internally. This, however, is not in accordance with Qi Gong, which requires us to have a commensurate sinking sensation, ensuring balance and root. In our daily lives this can bring about a new awareness of functional efficiency and pleasure in our internal sensations.

In Qi Gong the upward movement of the arms would be preceded by a distinct thought to initiate that movement. When the muscles receive the instruction and you can sense the initial movement, then it is possible to lead the movement, by thinking it. In the Qi Gong community it is referred to as 'the thought leads the Qi', in other words, 'think it first'. Energy is activated in a particular area, and then motor neurons fire to begin the action and energetic resources immediately become available. Next, as the hands are rising, consciously create the downward sinking sensation internally and in the muscle, even those that are activated. As the hands rise further and the muscles and ligaments around the joints tighten, try to relax them consciously and let the joints pull 'open'. Once the hands are high, let the elbows rotate inwards slightly, so that they are not artificially rotated out, and then ensure that the head is pulled up and the shoulders feeling a sinking and an opening of the joint.

After some practice it is possible to feel and understand that it is not just the shoulder muscles lifting and supporting the arm, but the whole of the internal connective structures, taking the weight and distributing the forces throughout. Devoid of excess muscle tension, the sensation of movement and awareness of gravitational pull is distinctly different than if we are constantly using localised excess tension to maintain movement and physical integrity. This is the 'sinking' (Song Jin) factor, and it makes a lot of difference to our entire perception of our physical self and our mobility. In fact, it is as if we have discovered a totally new sensation, which of course is not true, but we may have forgotten it since our infant days, when just standing up was a thrill.

Finally, the sensation of sinking and simultaneous rising has an apparent meeting point. It is at the fulcrum where all the forces on and in the body are reconciled, and that is the Lower Dan Tian located in our deep abdominal centre.

Finding the field

Traditionally, the Qi Gong community identifies three key important energetic centres in our body. They are all referred to as Dan Tian or 'Elixir Field'. One is located between the eyebrows and deep in the brain (Upper Dan Tian), the second is located behind the sternum, approximating the position of the heart (Middle Dan Tian) and the last (and the only one that we are concerned with here at the basic and intermediate level of Qi Gong) is the Lower Dan Tian, located deep within the abdomen. It is the place where our pre-birth life Energy or vital breath (Qi) can be most readily felt, nurtured and stored. It is fundamentally related to the seat of pre-birth Essence (Jing), considered to be pure generative and sexual Energy. It is the place where gross pre-birth Essence and Energy (Jing and Qi) can be refined to a subtle and pure energetic state, stored and mobilised. It is like an energetic battery. Finally, it is sometimes referred to as the 'furnace', or the place where the 'water' nature of pre-birth Essence and Qi is brought into a harmonious relationship with the 'fire' nature of post-birth Qi through an alchemical Yogic process.

The process of working on the Lower Dan Tian is a process of purification, refinement and transforming of the coarse to the subtle. This is the fundamental energetic work of Qi Gong and is the beginning of balancing and harmonising body, mind and Spirit (Jing, Qi and Shen). This is a long process that generally passes through distinctive phases of practice and cultivation and a growing awareness of the Qi Gong state. In traditional Qi Gong communities the eventual goal would be the transformation of Energy (Qi) to 'Spirit' (Shen) and thence to the pure state of the Dao, referred to as 'returning Shen to the void'. Don't expect this to happen overnight!

The Qi Gong process almost always begins with postural, respiratory and mental work. Beyond posture and breath, focused awareness for the most part is directed to the area of Lower Dan Tian, at least in the early stages. There are complex and obscure classical Chinese religious and medical explanations for what goes on here, but the sensed reality developed through practice is that the Lower Dan Tian becomes a field of awareness, certainty (firming the centre) and Energy at our very core. It is the apparent meeting point and fulcrum where all the forces on and within the body are reconciled, and through which the cohesive integrity of the body can be felt. It is a place where a deep, confirmatory experience of our 'life Energy' can be experienced and where our connectivity to the Earth is most evident.

Much of Qi Gong practice requires us to concentrate our mind on this to gain awareness of our physical centre. This allows us to generate a sense of enormous strength and firmness at our centre. Building awareness of this core changes our physical sense in movement and in our daily activities. We feel somehow more in accord in our actions and movement; more present and in ourselves. Building Lower Dan Tian awareness creates a conscious centre for the external forces we exert. It is a point where downward, upward, outward and inward forces are reconciled and directed, as well as a deep energetic root through which all aspects of integrated movement are internally connected, like threads drawn through the eye of a needle. Generally associated with the 'pre-birth' Energy and approximating the site of the umbilical connection, the Lower Dan Tian is the somatic centre of our being. Our mental and emotional connections with this area are also powerful, but they are slowly disassociated as we grow up and take on the mind–body dualism typical of Western culture. It is to our advantage to recover this connection, for ancient Chinese wisdom tells us that this is the place where the 'fire' and 'water', our Yang and Yin Energy, can be brought into harmony. Rather than allowing them to separate through our propensity to disperse and squander our life Energy, we are told by ancient wisdom that here is a critical centre of an inner cosmos where our life Energy can be brought under control and then refined and nurtured through self-cultivation to restore our health and vitality, and possibly Spiritual fulfilment.

Lower Dan Tian is not a specific location within us but, as the name suggests, it is a field or an area. It is often associated with a point just below the navel, a few inches inside the body, but it is best to see it as a broader area stretching from the front, below the navel (Qi Hai or Guan Yuan) to the back (Ming Men) and all around the waist. However, familiarity with Lower Dan Tian does give a feeling of greater density towards the centre of the field, rather like a ball. The line from Bai Hui (top of the head) to Hui Yin (between the legs) passes through all three Dan Tian, and lining up the three Dan Tian is a key starting point in both postural and Energy work.

Cultivating and firming the sense of Lower Dan Tian in static posture is generally the basic starting point, but you must also maintain awareness in movement. Think of Lower Dan Tian as a large ball that sits at the centre of the bowl of the pelvis. Its tendency when moving naturally is to seek rest at the lowest central point, and this will be our natural midline with a lowered centre of gravity. The slowness of movement associated with Qi Gong and Taiji alike should be thought of more as evenness of movement. In other words, once the centre has been established, evenness of movement must be adhered to, to train the centre to stay constant. Eventually it will be possible, as in Taiji boxing, to move fast and to keep the centre still. Once this feeling is established we will feel a link upwards to the centre of the chest behind the sternum, generally considered the Middle Dan Tian, continuing upwards to the Upper Dan Tian in the middle of the head. (This is the Central Energetic Channel.) These three Dan Tian are all considered as the locus of Energy (fields) and the aim of Qi Gong is the balancing, connection and integration of all three. Their connection is important and features in various methods of training.

The cultivation and practice of this essential link is a process of transformation, restoration, rejuvenation and clarity. In addition the Upper Dan Tian is associated with 'Heaven', mental and Spiritual (Shen) cultivation, the Middle Dan Tian with the post-birth Energy acquired from food and breath and our connectivity to sentient beings, and the Lower Dan Tian with the 'Earth', pre-birth Energy and Essence and our inherited constitution. Their connection is not just to do with balance and integrated movement, which is the gross postural aspect; on a subtle level it is to do with blending and transformation of Energy.

To begin with, the most important is the Lower Dan Tian. To cultivate and firm this centre is not so easy, and requires us not only to build a conscious awareness of this area, but first to create the physical conditions that generate the feeling, and then to cultivate that feeling. The feeling of the centre resulting from practice is tangible, and regardless of theoretical explanations or intellectual rationalisation, the sensations resulting from practice are what counts.

Postures to practise Lower Dan Tian awareness are varied in Qi Gong, but the simplest is just to stand. It offers the best opportunity to connect with all three Dan Tian, but especially Lower Dan Tian. Standing the simple Qi Gong way requires the feet to be shoulder-width apart and parallel, the knees to be slightly bent and aligned with the feet, the tail-bone to be tucked under slightly with the slightly rotated pelvis, the head to be pulled up and shoulders and chest relaxed. The arms hang by your sides naturally, with the armpits feeling slightly open as if you have two small eggs there.

The breath (Qi) should feel as if it is inhaled down to Lower Dan Tian. To do this you do not completely fill the lungs, but inhale as if you are filling from the bottom up (but do not fill to capacity). The diaphragm pushes downward and the abdomen expands comfortably. Breath should feel as if it has reached Lower Dan Tian. Obviously, breath only enters the lungs, but through abdominal breath the diaphragm extends downwards, elongating the lungs and creating a sensation that extends down to the kidneys and internally, deep into the centre of the pelvic bowl. The kidney area should feel as if 'grasping' the downward pull of the lungs. It is the sensation of breath meeting the Lower Dan Tian, compressing the abdominal cavity and creating a distinct sensation of hydraulic pressure. Simply standing is the fundamental Qi Gong and can be practised in our normal daily routine. The key, though, after posture and abdominal breath, remains relaxation and mental focus on Lower Dan Tian.

Concentrating our mind at Dan Tian allows us to quieten the mental dialogue while bringing us into contact with a more subtle sense of our energetic and physical self. It establishes a place of sensation that seems both specific and body-encompassing. From this place we sense and can adjust and refine both our back and front, upper and lower body; each subtle adjustment of the angle of our limbs, or the rotation or opening of a joint, or the lengthening of our spine, seems to register here, giving us the sense that it is truly a psychosomatic centre. It is as if it is at the centre of a web of connectivity that spreads throughout our inner landscape, bringing all parts into a connected relationship, whether in movement or stillness. This connectivity has material reality in the relationship between the movement of the diaphragm and the internal functionality of the organs and liquid landscape, as well as the connective tissue that links, like an intelligent web, all the parts of the whole body into a structural yet fluid and flexible integrated system. When one part adjusts, all parts adjust, when stillness descends, everything endeavours to come to rest. The centre of this matrix is Lower Dan Tian.

Finding, sensing and building on this field is at the very heart of Qi Gong, and the benefits it can offer stem from this developed awareness. The simple ingredients are setting up the posture, relaxing, regulating the breath and focusing exclusive mental attention on this 'Elixir Field'.

Simply breathing

One of the single most beneficial skills we can develop in seeking to be healthier, happier and less stressed is to learn how to breathe properly. Of course we all breathe while awake and asleep, and we generally take this activity for granted. It is remarkable in that we can breathe involuntarily, as we engage in speech and the activities of our daily lives, and we can also adjust our breath and regulate it voluntarily. It is through breathing that we can most easily engage and affect our physiology and emotional and mental state. Many of us, however, breathe inefficiently and with too much tension, thereby wasting this remarkable opportunity to benefit our overall well-being.

We inhale air into the lungs, where oxygen is extracted. Oxygen is needed to burn food and release Energy. In addition, the action of breathing expels through exhalation the waste product of the living process, carbon dioxide. Oxygen facilitates all metabolic function and thus the maintenance of good health and functionality is harnessed to the act of breathing. Getting that oxygen into our system efficiently and expelling waste efficiently is a biological priority, so it seems strange that so many of us go through life without a thought for our breath until we become ill, or breathless from climbing the stairs, or suffer respiratory disease.

When we are young we breathe naturally and comfortably. The diaphragm descends, stretching the lungs with it, thereby increasing the surface area to facilitate gaseous exchange, most of which takes place in the lower part of the lungs, so that the process of getting the air deep into the lungs is an important business. In the natural breathing of a child the abdomen expands in conjunction with the descending diaphragm, sucking air into the lungs, and contracts with the exhalation, as the diaphragm returns to its original position. Breathing is naturally through the nose to warm and filter the air as a first line of defence against airborne infection or extremely cold air, which might damage or restrict the workings of the lungs. The child intuitively understands 'natural' breathing and is unselfconscious about the expanding abdomen. As we get older we seem to lose the ability to breathe naturally. Our lifestyle and the development of our muscles and posture seem to play a significant role in the way we breathe.

When we sleep, our body generally returns to a natural abdominal breathing. The best time to observe this is when we first wake up, since, by the time we have got up, eaten and caught the bus or whatever else, our breathing may well be more sporadic, and we may be into a habitual method of breathing that is restrictive and inefficient, acquired over years of poor respiratory practice.

Abdominal breathing is typified by a gentle rise and fall of the abdomen. It must not be forced. The inhalation and exhalation are long, fine and silent (like a fine line) with no sense of oxygen deficit. In a stationary posture this type of breathing is achieved through concentrating on relaxing the body, especially the shoulders, ribcage and abdomen, and focusing attention on Lower Dan Tian. The inhalation should feel deep into the bottom of the lungs, giving the sensation of firming Lower Dan Tian and activating the kidneys.

Advanced practitioners will feel an expansion all around the waist and especially over the kidneys, giving the waist a 'full' sensation linked to the downward pressing of the diaphragm. It is sometimes referred to as accumulating and condensing Energy (Qi), since the sensation is that. It is this type of breathing that is most desirable in the practice of Qi Gong. However, movement requires us to harmonise inhalation and exhalation with either a contracting and drawing-inwards movement, or an expanding, stretching-outwards movement respectively. It is natural, since the inhalation delivers fresh oxygen, giving us the feeling of gathering our Energy and preparing us for the exhalation, where we expend our Energy.

Think of how you might breathe if you were pushing something quite heavy. The internal sensation is that of accumulating and condensing Energy in the Lower Dan Tian and then expanding it throughout the body or to a particular place, depending upon the movement or the activity. The idea is to practise this relationship between external movement and internal breath, since it this combination that has proven most effective in circulating oxygen-rich blood and efficient functionality.

Generally speaking, most people in their adult life and old age habitually use restrictive thoracic breathing, where the diaphragm is held rigid and the chest expands by virtue of the intercostal muscles. Combined with a rigidly held abdomen, the result is both costly in terms of Energy expended on the breathing, and inefficient in terms of oxygenation. As we get older and our posture loses its proper alignment and integrity, our breathing deteriorates. We lose muscle tone and our diaphragm often becomes restricted or frozen in its ability to draw the lungs down. In addition you will also lose the internal benefits of the massaging effects that the generous action of the diaphragm brings to the viscera and the glands located in the abdominal cavity.

Different modes of breathing can stimulate a particular mental and emotional response, and, *vice versa*, a particular mental or emotional condition can impact on respiration. Restrictive thoracic breathing, for instance, can bring on feelings of anxiety and mental agitation, whereas abdominal breath can bring about a more relaxed and tranquil mindset, crucial to the business of self-healing and optimising health and mental well-being.

The overriding strategy in Qi Gong is to bring about a high state of relaxation while the body is properly aligned, first, to reduce the mechanical stress and strain and second, to encourage, through relaxation, beneficial respiratory technique and the free and unrestricted movement of blood and Energy throughout the body. Much of Daoist health practice can be brought back to respiratory technique, especially when combined with focused attention on a Dan Tian, for instance. Inhalation and exhalation should be long, deep, silent, even and a continuous uninterrupted cycle. The result is replenishing, restorative and rejuvenating.

In Qi Gong respiratory technique the first and most basic level must always be with abdominal breath and Lower Dan Tian awareness. This is generally best achieved in a simple standing posture, as previously described, without the added complexity of movement. However, once it has been achieved in standing and the sensation and habit reinforced, it must be applied to movement. Obviously it is more easily applied when a set of movements have been studied to the point where you can begin to pay attention to the breathing without compromising the 'exactness' of the movement. It is an important level and brings what would otherwise be ordinary movement into the category of Qi Gong.

There is a note of warning though, and that is: sometimes trying too hard to regulate your breathing can disrupt it. It is often the case that when you are practising a set of Qi Gong and you pay excessive attention to your inhalation and exhalation, you may find that your previously calm rhythm becomes awkward. It is therefore important to be more of an observer than a controller. The golden rule is that the body must always follow the rhythm of the breath, rather than the breath being forcefully yoked to the movement. In all instances, though, the breath should feel natural and comfortable. It is the repeated and correct practice of movements with harmonised breath that eventually eliminates the need for respiratory rules.

In Qi Gong, and especially Taiji, some teachers do not advocate becoming conscious of the breath, on the basis that when the movements are performed correctly and the body is properly relaxed, then the breath will be naturally co-ordinated with movement. My teacher, Master Li, clearly states that without harmonised breath and movement there is no Qi Gong, so I believe that at the very least students must be made aware of their breath, and the inhalation and exhalation must be appropriate to the set of movements. Without being made aware of their breath they will not easily be able to adjust or refine it and so avoid continuing with what may be habitually poor breathing technique in their Qi Gong practice.

Finally, and although the abdominal breath is the primary breathing technique, it is important to note that the other key respiratory technique that it is important to be acquainted with is 'reverse breathing'. This is commonly associated with a Daoist meditational practice known as 'Small Heavenly Circuit' (Xiao Zhou Tian – explained more in the following section, 'Meditation'). This is considered to be one of the most important 'energetic' practices from the Daoist meditative arsenal. Reverse breathing as used in meditation is typified by a slight pulling in of the abdomen, starting from just above the pubic bone, on the inhalation, combined with a gentle tensing of the perineal diaphragm and a slight tightening of the anal sphincter muscles, releasing this on exhalation and allowing the abdomen to expand back to a normal state. Some Yogic practices are severe in this method of practice, but the rule of 'natural and comfortable' must be applied to it, since its effects are powerful and possibly damaging if overdone. Typical problems occur in uneven or jerky transitions from inhalation to exhalation and exhalation to inhalation, often accompanied by a sense of oxygen deficit and with consequent discomfort, stress or anxiety. In the natural method of abdominal breath it is much easier to overcome any 'jerkiness' in the action of the diaphragm and muscular resistance. Consequently, I believe the Small Heavenly Circuit, or at least the 'reverse breath' technique, should always be learned from an experienced practitioner and not from a book.

There are also other methods of breath regulation practice and differing approaches concerning which is best for what, but healthy abdominal respiration remains the most important to cultivate for both health and meditative practice. Even here, though, there are levels of attainment. An advanced level of abdominal breathing is referred to as 'embryonic breathing' and this, though perfectly natural, is considered a mature level of achievement. It is an example of recovering through practice a naturally occuring state that has been buried or forgotten. This is representative of the strategies and deep meaning of Qi Gong.

The aim of breath regulation is to harmonise 'inner' and 'outer' and to cultivate, accumulate and mobilise energetic resources and movement. It is also a strategy to still the mind, 'open' the body and dissolve deep tensions within the body matrix.

In martial practice, the long slow form cultivates basic abdominal breath, but this is not the case in the fast form or martial application, where accelerated explosions of Energy (Fa Jing) and a changing rhythm and pace, stamping and jumping as well as high kicks, require a technique that is based upon abdominal breath but includes a compression phase on the exhalation that allows the body to project Energy outwards. Fast forms are also typified by the combining of hard and soft, fast and slow, and the functional need of the movements (martial meaning) determines the use of the breath. At this stage of training good respiratory technique is natural and easily adjusted to the requirements and characteristics of the forms and methods of movement. The key is to build up the respiratory capacity and the efficient usage of energetic resources. In this way a fast and energetic form does not need to leave you depleted and breathless. When the breath is right, energetic movement is comfortable and change is managed easily.

Breath regulation is complex and technical, and so the primary rule of thumb, if in doubt, as in all Qi Gong practice, is be natural and comfortable and not to exert yourself to your maximum capacity. Breathing should bring about a commensurate sense of absorbtion and vitality, and not deficit or exhaustion. In general the qualites of respiration that are necessary to cultivate are: tranquil, slow, long, fine, deep and even. These are really natural qualities, and so the more 'natural' you are, the more these qualities will be restored.

Meditation

Meditation cultivates the higher levels of consciousness (Shen) and in my view is the highest peak to climb and the ultimate achievement of Qi Gong. Meditation is a natural progression in the Qi Gong journey.

As humans we possess a powerful sense of self, and we are therefore prone to viewing ourselves as independent and autonomous. We are critical, acquisitive and deterministic and we view the world and all that it is as something somehow separate, as 'object' to our 'subject', thereby affirming a sense of separation or removal from the world in which we live. The Qi Gong community sometimes refers to the idea that when we are born we are separated from the pre-natal 'vital force', 'original nature' or 'life force', and as such we live out our lives in a kind of schism, removed from knowledge of our 'true condition', disconnected from original Energy (Yuan Qi). Qi Gong seeks to reunite that which was separated and in so doing reveal our 'original' or 'true nature' and bring us into a resonant awareness of the Dao.

In keeping with Daoist thinking, intellectual analysis of our state of being and volitional deterministic action are all traits of the ego and lead us further from our 'original' or 'natural self'. The key to recovering this 'self' resides in the subconscious, where the imprint of our growing, pre-birth consciousness can be found. Intellectual thinking and the illusion engendered by belief in a deterministic material and rational world all conspire to separate us from the Dao. It is only through direct, intuited experience that we can reconnect ourselves with this universal, unifying ground, since its realm is beyond language and intellectualising. Dissolving the 'I' and dissolving the distinctions of 'subject' and 'object' by sitting in contemplation is the technique prescribed to bring about the natural emergence of the original uncorrupted and unified field of consciousness.

We all know that in our modern world it is difficult to get by without a degree of intellectual analysis and deterministic and volitional action. In addition, our 'ego' is our tag which defines us and proclaims who we are in a world that demands we are somebody. Society is an entity against which we are taught to see ourselves and by which we are influenced and judged. We are continually under pressure to achieve material success and social status and engage in a lifetime of work, the results of which are often hard to see beyond material gain. However, it is possible to find within ourselves a sense of a bigger picture, a greater reality, against which we can view the mundane ebb and flow of our lives, and although we must live in the world that we all conspire to create and believe in, we can also intuit a deeper, unifying and transcendent principle.

The strategy to achieve this is to quieten the internal dialogue and the streams of thoughts that normally arise. To facilitate this it is important to close down the senses ('thieves') and to calm the emotions ('hooligans') and look inwards. This means to take no notice of sounds and sensations that surround you. You do not want anything that the attention can hook onto to distract you from your purpose of closing all the gates and darkening the house. Habitual mental activity will rebel against this and assert some sort of internal dialogue. The mind is used to constant stimulation, unless sleeping, and it will try to recover its normal activity if the preferred type or amount of stimulus is not available. Meditation is consequently very difficult for many people, who are more used to allowing thoughts to roam freely. We are used to this and it brings us comfort, since it reinforces our sense of self and engagement with the material world. Training the mind is like a mother trying to teach an infant to sit still. The child is easily distracted and fidgety.

It takes some time to be able to quieten our habitual mental need for distraction and stimulation, but perseverance will increase the time you can sit with focused attention. You notice when thoughts arise and allow them to dissolve without following and prompting them. Stillness comes when you no longer indulge in the thought game, and although thoughts may continue as internal chatter, with practice they soon dissolve, since they lose their value without a supporting and relevant context. There is an affinity between the succinct and clear, fluid movement of Qi Gong like Taijiquan and the quality of stillness, or the depth of stillness you have achieved.

When the internal process of Energy cultivation has been refined and Energy is abundant and circulating freely throughout the system, optimising health, then the ground is fertile for subtle Energy to cultivate the refining and distillation of mental activity and consciousness to a subtle level, which is sometimes described as 'returning Spirit to the Void'. This is a transcendent state where 'nothingness' is directly intuited as the original, undifferentiated state of pure, radiant consciousness.

The process begins typically by cultivating and strengthening the body through stretching, postural refinement, opening the joints, lengthening the muscles and dissolving tension, followed by cultivating internal awareness and integrated movement. Third, through specific mental and respiratory practice, you cultivate, mobilise and circulate Energy, stimulating and balancing the energetic and physiological systems, and refine your practice so that all external movement and internal activity is guided and induced by mental intention. The prevailing condition at this point is a quiescent equanimity with a heightened awareness of the internal energetic landscape. Finally, and to go a step further, you direct that Energy through meditation to retune and refine consciousness. In Qi Gong, sensing and refining the energetic body is the means through which the goal can be achieved. It is the platform upon which a higher and subtle mental state is reached. The Qi Gong path is an awakening and a process that moves progressively from the coarse to the refined, and then on to more subtle levels.

After the years of study, all the forms, all the exercises, all the practice and all the theory, the need for meditation dawns as an inevitability. This is the nature of the process of self-cultivation.

In the same way that an artist may try to reveal the inner or true nature of mountains or bamboo by the sustained, sensitive and empathetic rendering of the subject, eventually transcending its mere visual characteristics and expressing its intrinsic nature, meditation naturally moves us on to a deeper level of self-cultivation, nurture and realisation. It is a difficult path.

Although all Qi Gong in a sense requires a meditative state of mind, it is important to realise that there are degrees and depths of this state. The deeper the state, the more beneficial. Meditation has the function of cultivating a deeply quiescent and relaxed state, and is sometimes referred to as 'entering stillness' (Ru Jing) or 'entering a contemplative state' (Ru Ding, a Buddhist term). The term Ru Jing also alludes to a deep level of 'real' stillness or state of meditative practice where the sense of self dissolves and the subject and object and emerging thoughts disperse spontaneously, without substance, like small clouds in a blue sky. There is no 'me' and no 'other' and the boundaries of physical self, conceptual thought and language dissolve into a state of pure awareness, pure consciousness. There is no longer a subject to meditate or even an object of meditation. This process can be likened to clearing the dust off a mirror to reveal the pure, original, uncorrupted state. It is a long process, since, to continue the analogy, the mirror continually gets dusty, but slowly and through continual and sincere effort the radiant brightness is revealed and eventually becomes sustainable.

To a certain extent all meditation means 'entering stillness' and all meditation aims to 'dissolve' the construct of self or ego. Ru Jing though is both a stage, a goal and a process, and it is in its simplest sense the attainment of a quiescent mindset, free, or at least unattached to internal dialogue and the distraction of the senses. It is a basic requirement of all Qi Gong practice.

Another method to achieve a transcendent stillness is sometimes referred to as 'guarding the one' (Shou Yi). In its simple sense it requires the practitioner to focus attention exclusively on a point on, or in, the body. Lower Dan Tian is a common point of focus, though Upper Dan Tian also figures significantly in Spiritual Qi

Gong meditation. Shou Yi is a comprehensive practice it is based upon cultivating a lifestyle and habits of conservation and purification that keep attention firmly and permanently on the Dao, creating a fertile ground for a transcendant realisation.

Guiding internal energetic currents through the body is an advanced level of meditative and medical Qi Gong, as is Energy absorption from external sources (trees, sun, moon, stars, etc.), and this level is mostly suitable for the more mature practitioner. These methods are all employed across a wide range of Qi Gong meditation and all serve their purpose in cultivating, replenishing, mobilising and distributing Energy, as well as directing Energy for healing. The overriding emphasis, however, must be on cultivating a deep sense of stillness and a clear, uncluttered mindfulness, and this remains true for all levels. There is a direct relationship between the quality of stillness and the effectiveness of your practice and its value in daily life.

The many forms and sets of dynamic Qi Gong are designed to promote specific health benefits or martial ability, but the higher levels of still Qi Gong are a new challenge for those who are accustomed only to sets of prescribed movements.

Although much 'still' Qi Gong is practised in a standing posture, meditation is best practised in a sitting posture, since there are fewer demands placed upon the body than when standing. This allows for a fuller relaxation and full attention on the internal mental work. The Lotus posture is considered to be the most stable, since it provides a three-point triangular base maximising stability. However, not everyone can do this, and indeed for some it may cause discomfort and stress, which is far from being conducive to meditation. Never force anything – it is contrary to the guiding principles of Qi Gong. Simply sitting on a chair or stool is fine, preferably on one that is the right height off the ground for your size.

The most common form of still sitting meditation is the practice of the 'Small Heavenly Circuit'. This is a most important level to achieve and is a doorway to deeper Yogic practice and health maintenance.

The purpose of meditation in Qi Gong is both medical and Spiritual, and this is true of the Small Heavenly Circuit. According to the traditional Qi Gong community and Chinese medicine, the 'Heavenly circuit' runs up the back (Yang), over the head and down the front (Yin), reuniting with the Yang between the legs at Hui Yin. Yang and Yin Energy are linked in a circuit and act like energetic reservoirs to fill up areas of depleted Energy deep within and throughout the body. In the Small Heavenly Circuit mental activity or intention leads (Dao Yin) Energy up the back channel by thinking the path. Energy is activated by directed thought, and once the mental path becomes hardwired, the sensation of movement along the path is palpable, like a pulse or a flowing stream.

The ability to mobilise Energy in the Small Heavenly Circuit also means that you can further your practice by raising Energy through the spine and also up through the central line of the body into the brain. These additional roots are natural extensions to the achievement of the Heavenly Circuit, and serve to clear energetic stagnation in the spine and brain and the key pathways of the Energy matrix. There are many meditative practices for building energetic awareness within the body, as well as dissolving blockages and energetic distortion.

Qi Gong theory states that the small Energy circulation brings about what is referred to as the Yin–Yang reversal, best represented by the Daoist illustration of a sage whose Lower Dan Tian comprises a cauldron of steaming water set over a fire. It symbolises the union of pre-natal and post-natal Energy, represented as water and fire respectively. The downward flowing propensity of the cool and refined Yin pre-birth Energy (associated with the kidneys, Lower Dan Tian and water) is brought into a functional relationship with the upward rising propensity of the hot and coarse, Yang post-birth Energy, associated with heart and fire.

The metaphor indicates that, left alone, the fire Energy and water Energy would inevitably separate, water flowing downward and fire rising up, bringing about the loss of energetic cohesion, ageing and ultimately death. In the Small Heavenly Circuit Qi Gong seeks to draw down and cool the coarser fire Energy of the Middle Dan Tian and post-birth Energy, and bring it into harmony with the subtle Energy of the Lower Dan Tian. It implies a reassertion of the energetic and functional relationship of pre- and post-birth Energy and the rejuvenation of our energetic resources. However, metaphors, especially ancient ones, are multi-layered and the idea is much more complicated than this simple working explanation implies.

The imagery is profound and poetic and has enormous value in medical and and alchemical Yogic Qi Gong theory and practice. The method of the Small Heavenly Circuit is designed to reassert and revitalise our energetic core and store and distribute Energy throughout the Energy matrix. In a way, this meditation slows down our propensity for 'burning up' all our life resources and therefore serves to prolong life. Consequently, it is is a cornerstone in the art of achieving longevity and Eternal Spring.

The deep stillness, openess and relief that are experienced in meditation relieve our whole body of deep tensions and stress that are the residue of our life to date. Meditation is healing rest. It is different from sleep, since the mind is fully intent on a single point, path, or inhalation and exhalation of breath, or simply on listening internally and witnessing its own activity. It is attentive in an unself-conscious and unstressed way, listening and feeling in the moment unattached to the thoughts that arise in an attempt to recreate our normal habitual levels of mental activity. Meditation is the means to stop the leakage and dissipation of our life Energy. It is the method of looking inwards and cultivating more subtle energetic paths and higher states of consciousness.

The practice of meditational Qi Gong must be undertaken without any real concern for the outcome. It should not be a goal-oriented practice, or intellectualised, and the benefits and realisations that arise from practice should emerge naturally. Obviously it is best practised in a quiet and conducive environment, without undue external distraction, but I have found that any opportunity should be taken to look inwards, shut down and 'darken the house'.

CHAPTER 11

Mobilising Energy

Forms

Most Qi Gong, including Taijiquan, works on both 'external' and 'internal' elements, with the internal elements being the most important, though achieving them is contingent on external requirements. Dynamic Qi Gong practice is the practice of special 'forms' or sets of movement that are designed to accumulate and mobilise Energy to bring about a balanced physiological, energetic and mental integration. All Qi Gong comprises regulation of body, breathing and mental activity. Some modes are more inclined towards the first two regulations and some the last two.

Qi Gong forms generally involve slow, gentle movement of the arms, expressing a full range of mobility: extended or contracted with rising or falling, opening to the side, one pulling and one pushing, one lifting, one dropping, etc. – in other words, the full range of possible movements, encompassing also rotational capacity. As well as standing postures there are also stepping forms where the weight is shifted from predominantly one side onto the other. In most instances the torso is generally held erect so as to create an easy sense of balance. Many Qi Gong sets can, however, be done sitting, and some even lying. These are particularly important in medical Qi Gong where practice is part of a recovery programme and standing may be medically prohibited or physically impossible.

Qi Gong movements have special characteristics. Movement generally follows the rule of minimal exertion to achieve the shape, and consequently minimal stress on the body. You should not expend so much Energy that you feel depleted after practice, and neither should any movement be forced beyond your comfort zone. Learning to moderate movement and the exact amount of Energy expenditure is a long process of refinement.

Rotational movements in the arm should never be forced beyond what is comfortable and joints should never be locked. Movements should barely press on the boundaries of your normal mobility, but you should also intend to increase your range of mobility. This is the cumulative effect of regular practice over a long period. Extending and contracting movements in the arms should be circular rather than straight and incorporate a slight rotational, spiralling characteristic. Upper body rotation must be generated by rotation of the pelvis, but not so excessive that it compromises the structural alignment and load-bearing ability of the knees and legs. Any shift in weight must be done slowly, while recognising the point of stability and balance at each moment of movement (Zhong Ding).

The overriding principle is generally 'natural' and 'comfortable'. Combinations of movement work predominantly on different parts of the body and internal organs, as well as circulation of blood and Energy throughout the body. Qi Gong sets of movement aim to mildly stimulate and lengthen the muscles as well as 'unstick' connective tissue. They aim to restore optimum muscle length, tone and efficiency, as well as increase the efficiency of the connective tissue matrix. The slow movement of Qi Gong allows you to 'squeeze' or engage the muscles rather than overtly contracting them. Repetitive practice rehabituates the body to a new, less stressed and wasteful functionality, thus fulfilling the golden rule in Qi Gong, which is to conserve and cultivate Energy rather than expend it wastefully.

Dynamic Qi Gong requires you to use Energy to gain Energy, and finding the balance is a case of fine-tuning and experience.

Twisting, stretching and contracting movement combined with alternate weight loading on the legs increases bone density and stimulates blood flow and lymphatic drainage, while massaging the visceral organs. The spine is stretched and the controlling muscles, ligaments and connective tissue that sheathe the spine, connecting cranium to sacrum, are all equally and gently worked by Qi Gong movement. Many Qi Gong sets target specific areas of great importance to our general health and well-being, like the spine, or the liver, heart, lungs, spleen and kidneys (Wu Zhang – the visceral organs).

When the body is integrated and balanced in movement, respiration harmonised and the level of stress optimised, then the internal sensation of 'Energy moving' can be brought under the guiding control of the mind. This is a mature level and is the cumulative result of right practice and proper awareness.

Although all medical moving Qi Gong will follow the general principles of gentle and modest movement, many martially oriented Qi Gongs are more demanding. They require the body to hold or to repeat movements and postures for reasonably long periods. Obviously this ability needs to be built up over a period of progressive training. However, even then Qi Gong, assuming it is from the 'internal boxing schools', must simultaneously cultivate relaxation and internal 'sinking'. It is a very specific process and must be done carefully, otherwise it will result in excessive muscle power and hardness. At first this does not seem to make sense, but properly executed the results are clear to see and to feel in your own practice. If you are too enthusiastic and excessive, as many are when they meet martial Qi Gong, then it will be counter-productive.

Like all Qi Gong, repetition and the cumulative effects are the key. Excessive or prolonged sessions are counter-productive, since these will incline towards using pure physical strength and stamina rather than mental control and relaxed strength. This process, especially in the martial Qi Gong of 'internal boxing', is often referred to as 'refining steel'.

Martial Qi Gong aims to cultivate both Qi and trained power (Jin) by developing co-ordinated and integrated movement and rooting, as well as internal and external connectivity. The internal connectivity denotes the mind intention (Yi) leading Energy (Qi) which leads the trained power (Jin). External connectivity means various things, but most simply it implies the co-ordinative relationship between the hands and feet, elbows and knees and shoulders and hips. Taking into account internal and external connectivity, this is referred to as Liu He, the Six Principles.

Regarding the 'internal schools', the type of training that falls under the heading of martial Qi Gong trains the power of the whole body to be realised in an instant, delivered in an integrated and unified force, specifically directed. That trained force or integrated power can be expressed in ways other than just striking, and these are discussed in Chapter 12, which is devoted to Taijiquan as a boxing art.

All Qi Gong seeks to mobilise internal Energy and to refine the practitioner's awareness of it and its movement. The uninterrupted flow of Energy throughout the body is the process of self-balancing and self-healing.

External movements can serve to stimulate and guide Energy to various parts of the body for martial or medical reasons. They can also create conditions for external Energy to be absorbed and internal Energy (excess or distorted) to be expelled. Advanced Daoist and medical Qi Gong focuses more on the internal awareness and movement of Energy than on the external form, though external form is the starting place for nearly all Qi Gong practice. In some instances form can be dispensed with and thought alone can be used to circulate and absorb Energy.

In the West many students, especially those interested in the martial aspects, are keen to achieve a high level quickly. This may lead to overpractice in the belief that more is better. This is not true and will undoubtedly bring about imbalance, which is against the key tenet of Qi Gong – no excess and no deficiency. Certain Qi Gong, especially martial, can cause not only internal damage if not developed properly, preferably under good supervision, but also mental imbalance, excessive libido and feelings of being invulnerable and extremely powerful. As such it should always be treated with respect and caution, and proper guidance is necessary to practice these forms of Qi Gong. Generally speaking most forms of medical and Spiritual Qi Gong do not cause harm, personality imbalance or illness, though there are always exceptions. Excessive practise and obsessive interest should be avoided.

Taijiquan as Qi Gong

In China Taijiquan is now considered a Qi Gong as well as a highly respected martial art. Qi Gong, however, is not considered a martial art. Though there are many Qi Gongs that have been devised to support the characteristic fighting skills of the many martial arts of China, they do not generally comprise a fighting system on their own.

The reason why Taijiquan is so highly regarded as a Qi Gong is because the training methods and martial strategies comply with the essential principles of practice in most Qi Gong forms. The movements of the Taijiquan slow set require the practitioner to regulate body, breath and finally mind throughout a long series of movements that are based upon rotational movement, stretching and contracting, and shifting of weight, slowly and precisely. Integrated, harmonious and co-ordinated circular movements are the hallmark of the slow hand form of Taijiquan, and though the movements have martial function, the form stimulates both a relaxed, functional efficiency and the accumulation and circulation of Energy throughout the whole body.

In addition, Taijiquan is considered to be one of the internal schools of boxing. A prerequisite of the internal schools is the ability to 'relax' while cultivating correct martial forms, power and strategies. The training strategy for cultivating the Taijiquan is based upon a relinquishing of preconditioned body habits and reflexes (fight or flight) and it can be considered a process of unlearning or 'investing in loss'. The practitioner must undergo a strict re-education in body mechanics, movement, Energy awareness and cultivation, as well as the technical training of a martial vocabulary that is found in the various forms. This is all before embarking upon two-man sets designed to develop the characteristic martial qualities that define Taijiquan. This early building of the right Taiji body, mind and martial power (Jin) is really important, and without this achievement the later stages will not yield the best results.

It is commonly acknowledged that the internal methods of cultivating martial skills are slower and more difficult than the 'external' methods. It is also said that they have greater durability and longevity when they have been achieved, and in fact bestow good health and a renewed vitality in spite of age. It is also said that the external styles which rely on strength, speed and martial applications cannot be maintained into older age and at some point, unless they become internalised, ability and health may be lost or compromised.

Taiji is also considered a profound health practice because many of its most famous practitioners maintained their good health well into old age, living much longer than the life expectancy of their time. In Chinese culture this would be attributed directly to the regular, skilled practice of Taijiquan. Its reputation for good health, balance, mental clarity and robust strength and vigour into old age is without equal. It is referred to as 'Eternal Spring'.

Learning to walk and 'standing like a pole'

It is always interesting when teaching standing and walking step in Qi Gong, and especially Taiji, how difficult many people find it. This does not mean that they had it so wrong in the first place, since they evidently have the mobility to function adequately in the world, but bringing it within the sphere of awareness and bringing it under scrutiny changes significantly the sense of our mobility, co-ordination and balance. It also casts a revealing light on our posture and functional and co-ordinative skills.

When we begin to question our habitual mode of walking we are undertaking in our adult life an investigation of something we probably all feel we left behind in our childhood: upright mobility and learning to stand and walk. Qi Gong and Taijiquan training re-quires us to become particularly aware of our movement and posture and how we hold and balance ourselves. Qi Gong and Taijiquan all should start with an investigation into our standing and walking skills, since there is generally, by the time we have reached adult-hood, much that needs to be addressed in bringing both standing and walking into conformity with Qi Gong and Taiji principles. It is a conformity that has evolved to give us optimum health, comfort and happiness.

Standing is a chance to consider some of the alignment principles that we have mentioned in Chapter 10, and walking is a chance to apply those principles to movement and balance. Cultivating an awareness of postural alignment is less about forcing the body into a newly adjusted shape and more about building relationships be-tween previously disparate parts and slowly increasing awareness of both external (physical) and internal (energetic) components, as well as really beginning to feel the force of gravity and how it acts upon us.

Many people who come to Qi Gong have health issues and some of those health issues are exacerbated, or indeed caused, by postural and mobility problems. So in learning the postural principles of Qi Gong and Taijiquan, you must be careful and progress slowly, lest you exchange one problem for another. Forcing new body shapes can be damaging. Postural alignment must be both explained and demonstrated. Manipulating the student is also beneficial, but more important perhaps is the time spent on guided standing and walking practice. This establishes over time a clear idea of what exactly needs to be remembered and adjusted and allows for the experience of simple practice to lay sound foundations of awareness of alignment, co-ordination and balance. When the mind is able to hold the idea of a connected shape, then the shape arrives, albeit slowly. Generally practice should begin with standing, and stepping first without, and then with, arm movements. Both Qi Gong and Taijiquan use both forward and backward stepping. Backward stepping can present new and sometimes novel sensations that bring us directly into an awareness of our sense of stability and the relationship between our front and back.

Revisiting our standing and walking skills serves the purpose of addressing posture and co-ordination, and gives us an important opportunity to begin work on understanding stability and balance in motion. Qi Gong and Taijiquan aim to create an efficient and highly developed awareness of weight distribution and relaxed movement, driven less by excessive (and often over-compensatory) muscle tension, and more by ground force and smooth mechanical efficiency. Developing these skills is fundamental and comes first.

Fundamental to this idea of efficient functional mobility is developing relaxed, smooth and integrated movement and an increased ability to focus the mind on maintaining correct physical structure. Practice requires regulating the integrated relationship of the external physical components and the internal energetic components.

The main way of establishing the external co-ordinative skills is to maintain a sense of connection between the shoulder and opposite hip, elbow and opposite knee, and hand and opposite foot. In addition the vertical connection between the base of the torso and the top of the head must be asserted. Building this awareness creates a sense of integration in forward and backward as well as rotational movement. If you joined up these points diagramatically with elastic lines and moved about, you would see how the external elements of the body should be connected to retain a sense of cohesion in movement. In addition, you will very quickly see how, if you overextend or over-rotate shoulders and hips, you will lose that relationship, and hence lose your integration and possibly your sense of balance.

The internal energetic components are much more complicated and are often neglected, since they take some time to develop. They begin with the mind, or mental idea (Yi Nian) and the intention to create coherent posture and movement. The mind intention leads the Energy (Qi) to form the shapes and smooth and integrated movement. Constant practice refines movement and the elastic strength (Jin) that evolves from correct Qi Gong and Taijiquan practice. That relationship is described as mind intention (Yi) mobilising Energy (Qi) which supports the internal force (Jin).

Qi Gong and Taiji training must therefore deal with establishing these connections. It is obvious that the external connections are the best place to begin, and this can be done with standing and walking practice. More advanced walking practice in Taijiquan will incorporate martial movements taken from the slow form and repeated in forward and backward stepping, as well as more complex step routines. The primary purpose is to establish the connections and to cultivate the quality of Energy required to fulfil the movement, and eventually the right amount of power and stretch to achieve the fluidity. It is important to strengthen, tone and stretch the body appropriately (not excessively) and provide a vocabulary of specific movements that reflect function and/or stimulate the cultivation and circulation of Energy (Qi flow). The vocabulary of movement must become so habitual that it totally replaces previous habitual modes of standing and moving.

In simple standing (Parallel Feet – Ping Xing Bu) the rules of body alignment must be observed. Proper alignment must build an awareness of the downward gravitational force and the return ground force so that the vertical axis facilitates the distribution of weight efficiently downwards while allowing the efficient return of the ground force up. From this energetic experience we understand all our mobility and functionality. It is the context of our awareness.

Physical tension in the body creates resistance to the sense of 'sinking' that results from the efficient downward distribution of our weight. In turn the sense of the return upward force generated from the ground must rise up comfortably without hindrance. Your physical structure must therefore be appropriately aligned so that the forces within and on the body can be distributed effectively.

The skeleton should feel erect, as if pushed upwards in opposition to the ground, while the big muscle groups should feel as if they are sinking, pulled downwards by their own relaxed mass. This internal up and down sensation is important in establishing our 'centre' and our sense of being 'rooted'. It also allows the torso to drain tension and to be properly supported by the spine and seated on the 'platform' that is the pelvis. The challenge is to refine the integrating link between the torso through the pelvis into the legs and the feet. The proper relationship allows the joints and spine to be 'opened' and ligaments and muscle groups, particularly in the back, to be progressively stretched.

Simply standing allows us to cultivate an investigative inner awareness. It is an opportunity to simply stop, sense and cultivate our stillness and symmetry and feel the internal energetic climate and currents. We quickly realise that we can adjust this climate by simply standing, sensing and dissolving habitual tension. If we observe ourselves internally, systematically moving through our bodies (Fang Song Gong), relaxing the muscles and the joints and noticing areas of stress and tension, not only can we change our physical self but we begin to feel layered aspects of our very being and realise that we can change the inner climate for the better. Simply standing allows the undistracted awareness of our sense of being in space.

Basic standing is used for much fixed-step Qi Gong practice and is the beginning and end posture of all Taijiquan forms. Its natural simplicity also allows the opportunity to develop the directing mental intention that is required in much Qi Gong. Generally standing may be accompanied by the hands laid on top of each other over the external location of the internal Lower Dan Tian. Mental focus here combined with standing engenders a naturally relaxed and attentive feeling and awareness of Energy at our centre. It also puts us directly into contact with our three primary axial centres – Lower, Middle and Upper Dan Tian.

Because walking is more complicated and requires more physical exertion, it must be introduced slowly. Generally, stepping skills should be developed first, followed by hand–arm co-ordinated movement. Stepping or walking step practice in Taiji brings about integration of movement. It encourages a new awareness of our lower body mobilty and the pelvic link to the spine. It allows us to work on retaining relaxed alignment and horizontal stability when stepping forward and backwards.

When hand movements are added it is the beginning of building the connection and integration of upper and lower. Body alignment must therefore be in place, since otherwise most people find that they are trying to regulate too many elements. In addition when the hands are introduced, typically extending one out and withdrawing the other, with simultaneous advancing and retreating leg movements, we soon discover that waist rotation is also required. Waist rotation is the channelling and connecting factor between the lower and upper body. The shifting of weight forwards and backwards creates alternating return ground forces, amplified and directed by the leg–waist relationship and transmitted up the back. This Energy can then be distributed to either arm or to the hands. How the Energy is distributed depends on the mechanical and energetic integrity of the body and the unhindered physiological pathways, as well as the directing will of the mind. Only relaxed musculature and properly aligned structure can provide the right transmission and sensation of this.

Finally, everyone has their own measure in walking and in standing. For instance, some individuals may have a tendency to step too far, or assume too wide a posture. I have noticed that such excess may be related to one's self-perception and projected persona, rather than to one's actual size.

In Parallel Feet posture most people assume a stance wider than their shoulders, believing that it expresses their solidity and 'firm' centre, and in stepping they may step out so far that they put the body under stress. Conversely, some people may take a stance or a step that is not wide enough to reassure them of their stability. Your own measure must be the result of practice and ability. Critically, standing in Parallel Feet posture or stepping forward or backward should not mean compensatory movement in the spine or pelvis. This would be considered in Qi Gong terms to be unnecessarily demanding and requiring too much effort.

In stepping, the leg must be able to step out and withdraw without committing the weight of the body or compromising the stability of the head, spine, waist and weighted leg relationship. For most people walking is barely controlled falling. Qi Gong and Taijiquan walking teaches us to remain stable at all times (Zhong Ding) and never to compromise the stability of our centre by rashly overextending our step and falling uncontrollably forward. This also applies to extending the arm and hand movements.

All movement must be judged by its relationship to the 'stable centre' and the integrity of the posture, either in fixed step or in motion. There should be no excess in movement and also no deficiency. This can help us achieve the perfectly balanced movement. The reduction of excess stress and strain in our body is a major strategy of Qi Gong and Taijiquan. In achieving the truly balanced state and all that that entails, we are able to maximise our mobility and functional potential. In addition we are able to calm our mind and facilitate the use of our mind to direct our posture and movement.

Qi Gong uses walking and fixed-step practice and it is this fixed-step practice that offers us one of the simplest Qi Gongs both for health and for martial training. It is commonly referred to as 'Pole Standing' (Zhan Zhuang) and is a standard practice in Taiji training. It is worth mentioning this because out of all the Qi Gong systems its simplicity and effectiveness in both cultivating and maintaining health and in developing martial power and coherence is profound.

'Pole' or 'Post Standing' has a long history and there are variations of it in many Chinese martial arts. In martial arts training the postures can be held for a considerable length of time, sometimes an hour or more. In many systems, the depth and size of the posture might be considerable, and over an extended period this becomes extremely stressful. The size of the posture can be the clue as to whether the training strategy is primarily oriented to 'external' or 'internal' martial arts, or for health practice only.

Generally the posture is parallel foot stance and the legs can be more or less wide apart, the centre being low or high depending on the strength of the legs and the purpose of training. This Qi Gong requires a very strict adherence to postural alignment and internal connectivity and the opening of the joints and lengthening of the spine. From a health point of view all aspects of the posture must be modest so as not to put too much strain on the legs, torso and arms.

Zhan Zhuang is really based on simple and at first symmetrical arm positions, and this puts the body under slight amounts of stress. In holding those postures for a specific duration the mind can focus on reducing the level of stress felt and the amount of Energy expended to achieve the form and the duration of standing. In addition, standing in these postures gives you the opportunity to explore your symmetry and the distribution effect of energetic movement internally. It allows you to train the natural breathing method while putting the body into mild tension, and to cultivate the paradoxical relationship between muscles in tension and simultaneous relaxation.

Zhan Zhuang also massages the internal organs of the abdomen and cultivates an energetic coherence throughout the body. Mentally it requires the exclusion of any distractions and the quietening of internal dialogue. Generally the mental state assumes a state balanced between awareness of the sensed physical experience and exclusion of external distracting influence. Zhan Zhuang unites the dislocation of the distracted mind and the incoherent mind as well as cultivating balanced energetic distribution.

Zhan Zhuang may have as little as five or six fixed and symmetrical arm gestures and that is probably enough for most people. As you might expect though, there are more stepping and asymmetrical arm postures too. This system of Qi Gong is both simple and comprehensive. It is an important method in training the correct mental and physical qualities of Taiji boxing, as well as a simple regimen for health maintainance.

Forms and more forms

The range of forms in both the martial arts and Qi Gong is enormous and bewildering. Most people learn what they find conveniently close to them and may stay with that. Some may seek out teachers for specific study and some may be lucky enough to find someone who has a deep knowledge of various boxing and Qi Gong systems. However, keeping it simple is a good rule of thumb. Practice is the key. Knowing a lot without ever practising what you know is not a good way to go: there will be no benefits. I have often been told in China that to know one form well is better than knowing ten forms badly. This means that it may just not be possible to practise ten forms enough to master any one of them.

There are many crossovers between the martial and the medical in China and many martial artists will have a knowledge of Chinese medicine, though not all doctors will have martial knowledge. Medical Qi Gong may utilise some martial forms, but they will be without martial meaning and will be used for their health-promoting potential alone, and much medical Qi Gong will be without any relationship to Chinese martial culture at all. Threaded through the different systems are the more Spiritual practices which often sit in both camps, the martial and the medical.

Knowing a small vocabulary of Qi Gong forms for different 'occasions' may not be a bad thing, provided you are able to practise them all to a reasonable level.

An ideal 'all in one' Qi Gong is one of the slow hand forms of Taijiquan. Generally you need to be acquainted with a Qi Gong that tones, stretches and strengthens the body. This is your baseline and it should preferably be a dynamic moving Qi Gong. If you practise a Chinese martial art, then there will be accompanying Qi Gong forms that are associated with it, and which will enhance your martial skills. If your martial art is of the internal school, then the forms will most likely also be partially medical in that they will promote good health and Energy cultivation. The movements of the internal schools and external schools may often be the same, but they are executed and targeted differently and to different effect. For those who do not practise any martial art the medical systems designed as prophylactic and tonifying forms are the best, since they work on the muscles, joints, ligaments, tendons and connective tissue as well as opening the Energy channels and cultivating healthy Energy distribution and balance.

In addition a set that specifically targets the five main organs of the body (Wu Zhang: the heart, spleen, liver, kidneys and lungs) is beneficial for investing in long-term health. Finally a still Qi Gong like the Small Heavenly Circulation is important. More advanced Qi Gongs that involve external Qi absorption require a very good foundation in the three regulations of body, breath and mind. The practitioner must be sensitised to a mature level regarding both the external conditions that are favourable to Energy absorption and their own energetic state. These methods include 'Heavenly' and 'terrestrial' Qi absorption to replenish and purify one's own energetic storehouse.

These Qi Gongs stretch the boundaries of faith for a lot of people, who may feel good from Qi Gong practice but fail to see how, or what, you might be able to absorb from outside yourself, unless it is in food or liquid. The methods generally involve absorption of Energy from shrubs and trees or from the sun and moon, or simply 'Heavenly Energy', 'terrestrial Energy' or 'atmospheric Energy'. Daoist Qi Gong specialises in Energy absorption and moon, sun and stars, as well as localised beneficial atmospheric Energy (running water, lakes, etc.) are all part of the broad sweep of Qi Gong practice and worth investigating. In a world where natural Energy may be interfered with and impaired by energetic fields generated by human activity, we need to consider very seriously the conservation of natural places and areas where we can have good-quality exposure to 'natural' Energy. Finding quiet places without any Energy pollution is important to Qi Gong practice and is an aspect that is becoming harder to achieve as our cities, parks and countryside become more polluted and energetically distorted and masked.

Qi Gong is about balancing the systems and these types of Qi Gong have evolved to circulate, replenish, refresh and accumulate, as well as absorb, certain desirable qualities. Any learned form or Qi Gong activity, though, needs to be practised diligently for several years for its benefits to emerge fully. All Qi Gong benefits are cumulative in that they are the result of repetitive and right practice, and this is also the same for Taijiquan, whether for martial or health purposes (as a Qi Gong).

There is a natural tendency, when we have achieved a technical proficiency, to do fewer repetitions on the basis that you know how to do that now, so you can move on to something else. Qi Gong does not work this way, and technical proficiency alone will not always reveal the benefits until it is hardwired and the body, breath and mental activity have been regulated and harmonised satisfactorily. In a sense, technical proficiency is a stage and may be considered the 'craft'. For it to become an 'art' you will need to get beyond that stage. Repetition, therefore, is a key in both refining technique and cultivating the right body and internal landscape to maximise the benefits, and also to take it beyond the ordinary limits of an acquired skill.

Too much Qi Gong practice, however, can cause problems and imbalance, creating a predominance of certain feelings or desires and/or discomfort and possibly illness. Moderation is the key to successful practice. However, too little will not bring significant benefits, so it is important to be sensible.

Practice brings its own rewards and if you persevere, practice will gain value within your personal context and you may begin to miss it when you do not practise. It does not take long to begin to enjoy the feelings during and after practice and it is important to realise that those feelings grow and change and become more refined. A simple Qi Gong form practised regularly is better than overly complex forms that you may struggle with. Qi Gong is about taking the raw and coarse ingredients and refining them to the subtle and pure.

Finally, do not learn too many methods, since it not only becomes impossible to practise them all, but it will also be difficult to understand them all thoroughly. There is no perfect form, only perfection through practice. Do not expect too much too quickly. It takes time to adjust the body, understand the breathing and fashion the right mindset to create the best ground for growth.

Practice

*P*rolonged practice has a significant benefit to our physical and mental well-being.

As a holistic practice it is important to work on all three aspects of the 'three regulations': body, breath and mental activity. In fact it is impossible for the beginner to do this while studying a form, since the early days are primarily centred on co-ordinative and physical (external) achievement of posture, shape and movement.

From the beginning, though, mental awareness and learning how to consciously maintain the correct posture and shape are important. Generally speaking it is not worth trying to understand 'regulation of breath' until body shape and external accuracy are achieved. However, since the practice of Qi Gong is a process of continuous refinement and the aim is to harmonise body, breath and mind, there comes a point where all three regulations must be linked and then the long process of mature and subtle refinement can begin. Awareness of integrated movement, harmonised with inhalation and exhalation, is really first base.

Generally body movement and harmonised breath are the easiest and a first level of competence. This can be achieved quite quickly with diligent and sincere practice, providing the teaching applies adequate focus and offers proper methods of practice. At this stage the mental involvement is primarily to 'police' the body alignment and to cultivate 'sinking' (Song Jin), the relaxed awareness that is the essential of all Qi Gong that seeks to nurture Energy (Qi) and cultivate health.

Once you have achieved a good standard of physical form, integration of breath and movement and the ability to maintain a relaxed awareness and shape, both in movement and stillness, then it is time to increase the emphasis on the next stage of Qi Gong, which is refining mental awareness and directing intelligence. Regulating and refining mental activity will determine the ultimate depth and success of Qi Gong practice.

At this stage the external shape takes second position to internal awareness and sensation, since the external shape is now informed by internal awareness and the sense of movement of Energy through the postures. This is a much more subtle level of achievement.

Through the methods of 'regulating' the body, mental awareness can be said to be nurtured from the very beginning, but this is not the level of awareness that is used to sense internal activity since it should be concerned with regulating the body posture and form only. It takes time and persistent practice to go beyond this level and to understand the components of Qi Gong and bring them into a proper relationship. From the first level of awareness required of Qi Gong practice, the mental state evolves naturally towards a less self-conscious, less physically oriented, directing mode of thinking. The more advanced level should focus on developing sensitivity and awareness of the energetic aspects of Qi Gong practice, which are felt as the changing sensations that result from movement and respiration. Recognition of those sensations in turn brings about a higher level of refinement and more fine-tuning of physical shape and movement. This level is particularly enjoyable because you start to sense the potential and meaning of Qi Gong and feel the pure beauty and sensory delight of a higher awareness integrated with physical movement and breath.

It is important at this stage not to pay too much attention or have too high an expectation of results. Also it is important not to jump this stage, believing that you have 'got it'. There are levels of subtlety and the work of 'internal listening' and not interpreting, analysing or explaining is important if the 'intuitive' rather than the 'analytical' mind is to be cultivated and, more importantly, if the flow of Energy is not to be hampered by inappropriate concentration or distraction. It is considered that disruptive thinking and over-concentration or excessive will power can create distortions of Energy and hence illness or mental imbalance.

The development of a higher level of mental awareness and the ability to listen to the energetic sensations of the body leads to the more refined ability of bringing the movement and distribution of Energy under the guidance of your mental intention. Although this happens to a certain extent all the time, cultivating the skills of Qi Gong requires us to take what is natural and put it through a refining process, developing those skills to a higher level and elevating a natural process to an art. Projecting an idea, an intention (for instance, raising an arm, or the idea of Energy accumulation at Dan Tian), enables us to progress from idea to actuality and to stretch the boundaries of our ordinary awareness.

This stage brings improvement to all aspects of our functionality, mobility and, which is important, our energetic self-governing and balancing (Yin–Yang) ability. Such advanced practice brings a heightened and tangible awareness of ourselves as a living entity; not the intellectual knowledge and mundane presumption, but a deep awareness of our 'vital Energy' and holistic nature. At this level, the door is open to more refinement, distillation and tranformation of the essential ingredients of Jing, Qi and Shen.

When we achieve this level we come to realise that we are not just a closed system (energetically), but that Energy constantly flows through our own system and from our environment. This can be both beneficial and destructive and learning how to guard our Energy and absorb beneficial Energy is an advanced state requiring maturity of practice and a subtle awareness. The internal equilibrium necessary to maintain optimum functionality is constantly adjusting in relationship both to our environment and to our internal climate. That process can be sensed and internal conditions for refinement and maintenance of our internal landscape become possible. Replenishment of our 'vital Energy' also becomes a very real option. From this comes the enchanting and desirable goal of 'Eternal Spring' or longevity.

Because Qi Gong makes us very aware of our environment and how different conditions impact upon us, whether energetically positive or negative, it teaches us to seek out the most beneficial conditions of nurture rather than negative and damaging conditions. It is a self-preservatory state that is not generally promoted in our modern commercial environment where business exploits weaknesses that encourage poor lifestyle and a commercially oriented health culture. In addition Qi Gong calms and subdues the propensity for excessive emotional responses to our condition and events, and in so doing reduces the emotional impact on us and allows us to maintain a clear and uncluttered mental house. This can be viewed as a sort of emotional detachment. However, I do not mean the inability to empathise, but more the ability to regulate the harmful effects of extreme or prolonged emotional states and involvement which can, according to traditional Chinese thinking, impact adversely on our internal landscape.

Curiously, calming the emotions through practice does not turn you into a 'cold' person. On the contrary, it allows you to feel comfortable within a good emotional range while leaving out the extreme reactive emotions that are so often the indicators or the cause of an imbalance. However, there are always times when we are caught out, for example by a sudden death, when emotional reactions are beyond our normal range and the sadness may arise quickly and stay for days, weeks or even years. At these times Qi Gong is a tool that offers us emotional respite, re-centres us and dissolves the stubborn residual tensions and damage held deep within body tissue. In turn, this reduces the 'internal' pressure and thereby precipitates a more natural, less retentive resolution of sadness and grief.

Qi Gong practice allows you to progress from the cultivation of physical stability to the realisation of mental and emotional stability. Cultivation of the 'still centre' is perhaps one of the most important results of Qi Gong, since the emergence of this state means a growing maturity of practice as well as a deepening affirmation of the Qi Gong experience. It also means that Qi Gong can impact on your daily life by calming excessive emotional response and maintaining mental clarity. The growing internal stillness establishes the ground from which good health and mental well-being spring.

The mental well-being of Qi Gong cannot be thought of as a state of permanent happiness; that would be naive. Neither can good health mean that you never get ill. Mental well-being may be more accurately described as a sensory awareness of wholeness within ourselves. You feel natural and comfortably calm. Consequently, you are less buffeted by the events that surround you. In addition Qi Gong sensitises you to changing conditions (Yin–Yang) and helps you to respond appropriately in a balanced way that conserves your precious 'centre', without which you would feel energetically dispersed (emotionally and physically) and easily knocked about. Guarding our centre and our Energy is critical to cultivating the long-term benefits of Qi Gong. Regarding illness, Qi Gong is not a cure-all. Its main role is preventative, but there is no doubt that Qi Gong practice encourages remarkable conditions of recovery and regeneration.

Achieving maturity and depth of practice means that Qi Gong has become an integral part of your life as if you 'rest within' its law. It is the law of balance within change. It is the achievement of the Taiji (Dao).

Advanced refinement means to study the minutae of movement, respiration and commensurate internal energetic sensations by training the inward-focusing and inwardly aware and guiding mental state. This stage is about 'thinking' the movement of Energy and thereby guiding and inducing the physical sense of it. It is about reducing the predominance of the external and realising the movement of the internal. This idea is extremely important and must be practised until the mental focus becomes the energetic sensation. It is the meaning of the Qi Gong adage that Qi and blood follow the 'mental intention'.

The actuality of Qi Gong must be cultivated through practice and not through a delusional state brought about by premature expectations or intellectual or physical arrogance. The knowledge must be born out of the practice and not assumed through book learning or being told. In addition, when the Energy is felt, focusing on 'it' too intensely will hinder progress and possibly cause an imbalance or distortion. The skill lies in the level of 'unattached' mental focus projected from a quiet and still mental state. This is where the difficulty lies, because without the correct mental activity the sensations and guidance of internal Energy cannot be accomplished or refined. Although this process goes on anyway, though generally unnoticed by most of us, the aim of Qi Gong is to take our 'natural' state and cultivate it to a higher and more refined level. It is necessary to have this intention or you would never begin the study, but to have too great an expectation will handicap progress. In Qi Gong practice it is best to be unassuming, without preconceived ideas. Just be aware and notice what happens, without explanation or too much scrutiny or analysis. Certainty, confidence, knowledge and achievement are born out of long and sincere practice.

CHAPTER 12

Taijiquan – Supreme Ultimate Boxing

What is the point?

So far I have talked predominantly about Qi Gong and it will be obvious that within that term I have include Taijiquan (the martial art), since the essential principles of Qi Gong and Taijiquan are the same and fall within the range of Chinese health culture. However, at some point, the path of Qi Gong and the path of Taiji as a boxing art must diverge, since by definition a boxing art means gaining ability in attack and defence – a goal that is not necessary for good health, longevity or Spiritual development, which are the primary aims of Qi Gong.

Taijiquan borrows its name from Taiji, the philosophy or theoretical framework that explains all things in terms of change. Change, according to the Taiji theory, is an immutable law. Change is the ceaseless and inevitable condition of all things. Materially that change is expressed as states of Yin or Yang and together they are manifestations of the Dao. It is said that 'one Yin and one Yang together are Dao' (Taiji). This relationship is an expression of change and transformation itself. Like balancing scales, a state of Yin must inevitably transform to a state of Yang, and *vice versa*, in an endless reciprocal process. Taijiquan is a martial system that seeks to understand and use the law of change and the strategies based upon the interdependent but apparently opposite aspects of Yin–Yang theory to defeat an opponent.

Stillness (Jing) and dynamic movement (Dong) are key attributes of the Dao (Taiji) and the boxing art of Taijiquan is the cultivation and practice of Jing and Dong as a martial strategy to exploit the law of change (Yin–Yang) and transformation. Taijiquan can be said to be the practice and understanding of Yin and Yang, both within our self and in a martial context. Taijiquan is the art of understanding and exploiting the potential of the interaction between movement and stillness.

The principles of action determine that there must be a balance within oneself between stillness, being the mental, emotional and internal state, and movement, being the external dynamic and transformatory state, at all times. Typically, this is achieved first in solo practice and then with a partner. This is the method of first, understanding yourself within the theoretical framework and second, understanding others through partner work. Partner work teaches many valuable lessons and Taijiquan has specific ways of working with a partner that allow you to study and practise the theory and the methods without necessarily studying how to fight. These methods are known as 'pushing hands' (Tui Shou) and can be a friendly, co-operative means for two people to work together to perfect their Taiji forms and increase their understanding of the principles underlying Taijiquan. Otherwise, they can be more combative and lay the foundation for attack and defence techniques and skills.

The value of this is in the interaction between the physical, energetic and mental condition of your partner and yourself. This engagement allows you to firm the skills of co-ordinated movement and balance and the 'still centre' that Taijiquan requires, and refine it in the face of interference from an external source (your partner and all his or her intentions and abilities). It puts you on the spot. In addition it teaches you how to divert or neutralise your opponent's force, while seeking an opportunity to upset their balance. In martial terms this means to seek a favourable opportunity to attack. In more civil terms it means you can learn the process of change and transformation and understand how to respond intelligently and appropriately while protecting your own centre, and so learn a powerful way of conserving and protecting your own 'vital Energy'.

Since the process of change and transformation is considered an immutable law, coming to terms with it and 'feeling' it as a physical reality has enormous advantages. It becomes a 'body' knowledge that helps to reduce the otherwise common stress response many of us have become used to in our daily lives. This all translates well into daily life, where conflict and stress are a daily occurrence, and engaging with a multitude of people, all of whom may have a different agenda and emotional output, is normal and generally wearing. Taijiquan's martial methods provide a defence against the wear-and-tear of our daily lives and teach us to yield to excess force and flow with the movement of Energy that is our daily life.

Many people who begin the two-man practice aspect of Taijiquan are often quite shocked at how anxious, cautious and guarded they are when engaged with another person in this type of context. This exercise is about investigating and exploiting the dynamics of balance, and feeling loss of balance is very disconcerting. At first people find themselves easily unbalanced and physically compromised. It takes a while to get comfortable, but what happens in 'pushing hands' practice is an expression of how we are in our ordinary lives and our interpersonal relationships. This practice can reveal our weaknesses and show us emotional areas and fears that we have not engaged with before. It shows us how our physical centre is inextricably linked to our mental state and our perception of ourselves. By learning to calm the mind, guard our centre and give up the anxiety brought on by this type of joint practice, we can cultivate a relaxed and intuitive means of engaging. We train ourselves to become calm and sensitive to change.

Beyond building the foundation for the martial techniques of Taiji boxing, 'pushing hands' functions like a therapy where both parties are physically and emotionally exposed while using a very controlled physical forum to mediate. Some people come with their own agenda and see it as a state of competition, expressing the need to win or dominate immediately, while some people retain tension and mental resistance as a state of guarded emotional self-protection. It is a fascinating practice and at least until Taijiquan skills have been gained it should be a practice of mutual co-operation, otherwise it can deteriorate into a shambles of competing egos, push and shove. This is not Taijiquan.

Obviously there are rules of play, and as in the form, posture and shape, relaxed awareness (Song Jin) and balance (Zhong Ding) in movement are all key ingredients. There are also specific techniques that are practised, all of which are based on the martial strategy of exploiting the dynamics of balance within ourselves and in our partner. Working on the physical aspect allows confidence to grow and fears and nervousness to be left behind as the technical skills develop. As you slowly develop your sense of being grounded and centred, confidence and courage develop naturally as original and often debilitating fears dissolve. This is both a healthy and a fulfilling transformation, and also has a knock-on effect in our daily lives.

All things considered, Taijiquan 'pushing hands' is an excellent exercise for examining both the technical and mental components that comprise our mobility, co-ordinative skills and balance, and for many people who study Taijiquan, this is enough. As part of a Taiji syllabus it functions to develop alignment, shape, balance, rooting and co-ordination, all of which express a physical comfort and beauty of movement. In addition the mental focus and the circularity of movement are enhanced by the physical knowledge of your own movement in relationship to another. To take this further, though, means first, to practise a range of 'pushing hands' skills both in a fixed step and moving step and second, to understand how to apply the martial applications in a way that is commensurate with the Taiji principles of movement and engagement. Crucial to that knowledge is the interplay of Yin, soft, diverting and neutralising movement, and Yang, harder, attacking and directed movement. In a nutshell, it means that when your opponent is hard or attacking, you are soft and yielding, and when his Energy is expended or diverted and dissipated or confused, his emergent Yin state enables you to immediately express Yang attacking Energy. Achieving this opportunity is at the heart of Taiji skills and fighting strategy.

Block, hit and kick

Taijiquan is the study of the dynamics of balance in yourself and your opponent. It means keeping your own balance and exploiting your partner's or opponent's to enable you to topple him. This is a sophisticated strategy that is defensively oriented. (It relies upon the opponent's commitment to an attack.) It is a skill that must be trained, since it is not in accord with our reflex responses or our general perception of how fights are won.

As a martial art Taijiquan holds that our natural strength is sufficient to seriously injure or kill, should the need arise. Developing additional muscle power is considered more debilitating than beneficial. Instead, Taiji players believe in developing a technical repertoire based on diverting, neutralising and returning the force that is aimed at them. Taijiquan exploits and enhances the natural rotational ability of the limbs and the waist. It trains a touch-perception of the opponent's intention and force. This allows interpretation and an appropriate response specifically matched to the opponent's move, hence his Yang action, my Yin response.

Anybody can achieve basic boxing skills of punching and kicking; indeed these are natural aggressive tendencies and as such are the most basic form of attack, which is generally considered to be the best form of defence. It does not require much skill, for anger is enough to fuel and prime the body for a violent exchange of blows, but though this is certainly martial, it is not an art. Taiji trains a much more sophisticated skill. In China, Taijiquan is considered one of the highest forms of boxing achievement, whereas the block, hit and kick methods are considered the lowest.

Learning a martial art is about harnessing the body's natural ability to move in certain ways, and cultivating specific usage and skills. Many martial arts train the use of the limbs by building muscle strength, stamina, speed and hardness and then adding martial 'applications' into the equation. This is generally achieved by attack and defence drills that programme the practitioner to respond to, or issue, an attack in specific ways: block and strike, kick, throw or take down your opponent in a hardwired combination of movements that are carried out with force and speed and fuelled by an aggressive and competitive mindset. It has proved very successful and is the preferred route of the military, and competitive and spectator sports. It also works on the street and is quicker to learn than the 'internal boxing' methods.

However, the Chinese 'internal martial arts' like Taijiquan develop an entirely different skill that does not use competitive aggression, neither is it built on the block, hit and kick technique. Instead it is based upon the ability to perceive and interpret attacking force and direction, then diverting that force from your centre in order to destabilise your opponent. To do this Taijiquan uses the rotational ability of the body to divert incoming force sideways, upwards or downwards, as well as the ability to draw force into your centre to dissolve it. It is a martial strategy that uses little tension, preferring to remain soft and pliable and responsive – the antithesis of what happens to us when we tense up for an aggressive encounter.

Much effort is put into training this approach, since it is necessary to retrain the normal response mechanism. For a closer analysis of how this works you need to read on, but it remains to be said that the skills of internal boxing are not commensurate in any way with the conventional notion of strength and martial ability and this is why Taijiquan has had little credence in the West as a martial art. If your knowledge is based only upon the 'big slow form' it is hard to see how it can be effective. Also it appears less dramatic and dangerous than the more conventional martial arts that exhibit power and speed and the punch, high kick, push and shove vocabulary that we are all accustomed to see in films. In the West there certainly seems to be a cultural preference for this more overt, 'external' martial style.

In China, however, the 'internal' arts are regarded as the logical achievement of a process that often starts with the more external skills and then internalises them over a long period. There are good reasons for this. First, learning martial arts would begin at an early age, maybe at the age of around six, when the natural mental and physical ability of the child suits the more immediate, and perhaps gratifying, punch and kick methods. Incredible and impressive skill can be achieved in these styles, notably by the Shaolin monks. However, at a certain point it becomes necessary to address the business of martial efficiency with regards to Energy conservation, as well as progressing to more refined and subtle ways of defeating your opponent. Generally what was more external becomes internal; power and action are generated differently. This is more suited to growing older, and perhaps wiser, where skill must supersede power and strength. The old masters were renowned for retaining their fighting skills into old age and this is probably because they practised the internal methods.

The skills necessary to make the internal arts work take much longer to develop since they seem unnatural, elusive and mysterious to begin with. By this I mean that in a violent confrontation the normal response, indeed the reflex, is 'fight or flight', an atavistic reflex reaction that floods your system with the adrenalin needed to maximise available Energy, shut down unnecessary function and prepare the body and mind either to fight for your life or to flee. It is an instinctive response designed for survival.

Most martial arts try to teach a vocabulary of movement and an intelligent and controlled approach to fighting. Through fitness and physical discipline drills and combat rehearsal, the fighter can achieve technical skills that are hardwired. In this way he can use the 'fight' part of the fight or flight response to capitalise on the amount of available Energy and aggression that is useful for defeating an opponent. The internal arts, however, take a very different view. They specialise in inhibiting the fight or flight response and training the interpretive intelligence of body–mind harmony to exploit the action and the centre of the opponent. This generally means waiting for an attack to be initiated and responding to the direction and force of it by going with it rather than 'blocking' it, using skill, not force, to dissolve and disrupt the opponent's aggression. This skill incorporates diverting, neutralising, listening and interpreting abilities. This at first seems a very strange and unnatural idea, but this is what makes the internal boxing systems an 'art', being fundamentally interpretative and not system-oriented.

Protecting your centre and balance, receiving, diverting and interpreting attacking force and exploiting your opponent's balance are complex strategies. They require a particular range of skills that at first are alien to us and feel awkward but once you comprehend and experience them, you begin to see their effectiveness as the natural result of a way of thinking and a way of acting that are on the one hand martial, but on the other a strategy for dealing with life's hurdles and cultivating the body, intellect and the Spiritual self.

Methods and strategies of Taiji boxing

Taijiquan is based upon the theory of Yin and Yang, and so Taiji as a Quan (fist or boxing art) is the comprehension and use of Yin and Yang to defeat an opponent. In boxing terms, this means first, understanding stillness (Jing) inside and movement (Dong) outside; second, understanding insubstantial (Yin) and substantial (Yang), and third, refining the sense of balance (Zhong Ding) and rotational skills in both receiving force (Yin) and returning force (Yang).

The starting point of the Taiji form is Wu Ji, or the state of emptiness. This is the beginning standing posture of the solo hand form known as Da Man Quan. It is the first level of achievement of the Taijiquan. From this still and empty beginning the state of Taiji is born. It is born of the intention to move and separate the 'external' physical and 'internal' energetic components that are our functional mobility. The stillness, however, must remain at our core as the mental state of quiescent and sensitive awareness and the physical state of deep but alert relaxation (Song Jin).

The Taijiquan 'form' is a comprehensive set of movements that exercises and expresses a comprehensive range of mobility that explores our functional potential in martial terms. Inherent within the vocabulary of movement and styled by the notion of continuous and fluid change are the alternating states of Yang and Yin, typically expressed as the interplay of outward, extending movements (including martial strikes) and inward, contracting movements, simultaneous upward and downward movements, and clockwise and counter-clockwise rotational movements of the pelvis (waist) and arms and hands. Stepping or stretching forwards movements and sitting back or withdrawing movements alternate in conjunction with the arms to create a dynamic exchange between the substantial and insubstantial. Degrees of change where weight is moved forwards or backwards and from one side to the other are of course in accordance with the intention and the needs of the form. Taijii is the study of harmonising the substantial and the insubstantial, Yang and Yin, simultaneously, as prescribed by the Taiji laws of martial engagement. Power generated from forwards and backwards movement of the legs is reconciled and transmitted through the waist and the area of the Lower Dan Tian, which provides balance and stability as well as transmitting martial power up the spine. The waist acts as a pivotal hub and also as a platform through which the variable weight loading of the body and arms is transferred down to the ground, just as return Energy is transmitted back up from the ground for martial usage.

The Taiji form is a remarkable piece of choreography, and each posture must be achieved in full within a continuous and coherent flow of dynamic movement. In movement the player must cultivate a sense of internal ease and quiet awareness of all the component elements of shape and change, and external movement must appear and feel natural and unforced, crucially reflecting internal comfort and natural composure. A mental thread keeps the movement continuous as you simultaneously 'imagine' realising power in different parts of the body, according to the martial meaning of the posture. To achieve this the player must investigate and cultivate the potential dynamic of each posture and transitional movement without expressing force. In energetic terms, within the language of Taiji and Qi Gong, the whole body is charged and full of Qi that moves in currents that support and propel the particular movements of the form. The martial Energy (Jin) which is the ability of the connective tissue, muscles, ligaments, tendons and spine to transmit, store and issue force is supported by Qi but guided by a focused mental thread that at any point can manifest the potential force held within the structure of the form. In the Taiji community it is said that Qi manifests itself in the harmonious and integrated movement, Jin manifests in the hands and Shen in the eyes.

Taijiquan movement is brought about by moving steps, with alternate backwards and forwards pushing with the weighted legs, alternating between right and left in fluid exchange of 'substantial' and 'insubstantial' weighting. The kinetic Energy thus generated is further enhanced by combining with the rotational force of the waist, which generates the Energy for the circles that create the variety of arm movement and rotational movement that is characteristic of Taiji. As the legs alternate like pistons, the arm and hand gestures also alternate, separating energetically in terms of rising and falling, pushing and pulling, lifting and pressing down, twisting and folding. The circular gestures typical of Taiji are always separated into Yin (soft, diverting and gathering Energy) and Yang (hard, returning and releasing Energy). In the solo form this harder, Yang aspect is not overtly expressed, but can be thought.

At any point the circular movement (Yin) that is the path of continuous and fluid exchange and gathering of Energy can be changed into a straight line (Yang), and this is the point at which the Energy potential held in the circular form can be released as martial Energy (Jin). This idea is expressed as 'the circle becoming the square' and is the potential inherent within the dynamics of the movement. In martial usage the square is hidden within the continuous changing circle, since the idea is that you can read your opponent, but he cannot read you. Devoid of discernible intention and difficult to locate (owing to lack of resistance), you become less of an opponent and more of a shadow that attaches to, and follows, the attacker's aggressive gesture and intention. You are Yin to his Yang. Strategically, it is when his Yang is spent that your Yang Energy can quickly manifest in attack. These aspects are the Yin and Yang of Taiji, and if they are not understood and expressed, the form may resemble Taiji, but is not.

Throughout the set of movements known as the form, one holds to stillness as a mental, internal state, and movement as an external state. Internally, calm intention arises from a still, focused and undistracted mind and this generates movement – not careless or unstructured movement, but movement disciplined by the rule of no excess and no deficiency. This is the balance of Yin and Yang. Movement is trained so as to refine efficient, functional capability and our mental potential.

At any one time in the practice of Taijiquan, the student must train a natural awareness in understanding the differentiation between that which is full, energetically charged and active, and that which is less full, energetically passive and less active. Between the two there are many states where the complementary aspects are used to create at first an overt dynamic and later, as skill progresses, a refined and subtle dynamic.

Understanding the changing state of the body in movement within our own physical constraints and under the downward force of gravity is the achievement of the solo form.

In the beginning of Taiji solo practice, you learn the shape and gesture and transformation of integrated movement, upper and lower body harmonise, left and right sides co-ordinate and body awareness grows. At first co-ordination may be poor and movement without harmony or fluidity. Through persistence and guidance, practice progresses to a more comfortable and natural integration, and a more unified movement emerges. Constant investigation and refinement is necessary to take this further, to explore your potential. The range of mobility required in forming the Taiji movement vocabulary must be studied closely, and developed over a long period. The sense of movement must be cultivated and the source of movement must be understood.

Studying solo practice is a long process and provides the theoretical ground and all the physical vocabulary necessary for investigation and refinement. The process passes from gross, exaggerated forms and poorly co-ordinated movement to a greater physical awareness and refinement of body and movement. It is the process of refinement that is the 'internalising' of the practice. As integration and co-ordination develop, and the body is relaxed within the constraints of the principles, the 'centre' is recognised, activated and finally 'firmed' and made real. Balance and 'rooting' are understood.

As form ability develops, less and less physical effort is required and a deep sense of natural and relaxed movement grows. Slowly the body is reprogrammed, movement and transition become smoother and easier; the sense of the ground root grows deeper and the 'drawing up' gives rise to a simultaneous sense of upward flow and downward sinking. Movement becomes the easy response and expression of mental intention. In this way the mind becomes the master and the body acts in accordance, and although the vocabulary of mobility is relatively simple, it does engage all the skills of mobility that we as humans use regularly, and some that we do not. Taijiquan is both a physical challenge and an intellectual puzzle.

The movements of Taijiquan are not arbitrary movements but are a martial vocabulary, all of which has martial meaning. Each movement and each transformation imply martial application (Yong Fa), and without this knowledge much Taijiquan form looks empty of content and devoid of intention. Other Chinese martial arts share a similar vocabulary. After all, and in accordance with our physical attributes as human beings, there are only so many ways that we can attack, and only so many ways that we can defend. The vocabulary of movement in Taijiquan, as in all martial forms, contains within it (sometimes hidden) everything necessary. So what are the strategies that make Taiji different?

Defining characteristics

The Taijiquan solo form teaches continuous, integrated and harmonised movement. It teaches that upper and lower body must be co-ordinated; that power comes from the legs and root (ground) and is directed by the rotational ability of the waist. In addition the waist determines the turning of the torso and hence the movement of the arms. The arms reflect the rotation of the waist and can therefore move in a rotational relationship to the waist. In simple terms this means the anti-clockwise turning of the waist pushes out the right arm and facilitates the withdrawing of the left, and clockwise rotation facilitates the outward movement of the left arm and the withdrawing of the right. The hands move outwards at a tangent to the circle of the waist.

In addition, horizontal arcing movement of the arms, where one hands pulls and the other pushes (coupled force), reflects the horizontal mobility of the waist, a very important focus of training. In the analogy of a bicycle wheel, the waist is the hub and the arms are on the outer rim. This analogy also works if the wheel was set to rotate on a vertical plane, with the hub still in the waist (Lower Dan Tian), but in this case the bowing ability of the spine and its connection to the pelvis become the source of vertical, inward circular movement, and outward rotational movement is born out of the lengthening of the spine.

The ability of the body to generate circular movement is natural and is exploited fully by Taijiquan as a means of diverting attacking force without using force. It is a trained skill, since normal mobility must be enhanced and integrated and the integrated rotational component understood.

Power is derived from integrated movement, resulting from the kinetic Energy (of moving forwards or backwards and turning, etc.) that is generated in the legs and transmitted into the upper body by the rotation of the waist, and the spine's ability to store and release Energy to the hands via the shoulder, elbow and wrist joints. These elements are the focus of much training in a Taiji syllabus.

Such training is considered Yin or 'soft' and seeks first, to train balanced and integrated movement and second, to 'train out' the use of excess force and tension. In two-man contact exercises there is an opportunity to understand how rotational movement can be used to divert and destabilise an opponent. In addition, it provides an opportunity to reprogramme the reflex tensing that occurs when our centre, and thus stability, is compromised. If this aspect is not trained, the end result cannot be described as Taijiquan. However, good training does not ignore the complementary Yang aspect (cultivating martial power – Jin). It is said that when the Yin has been cultivated, the Yang aspect will emerge. This means that when the body has become softer and more flexible and is able to feel how Energy can be mobilised and mentally directed, then the martial force can be developed.

Taiji training requires the muscles to be as relaxed as they can be, in holding a posture or during transition from one posture to the next. Minimal stress and strain produces Energy-efficient functionality. The mind must be 'still' or undistracted, attentive and aware and, critically, directing movement and direction by leading and guiding the form. You must 'think it'.

Practice must also concentrate on cultivating the 'softer' rather than 'hard' tense muscle force of 'external' styles. The Taiji classics talk about the soft overcoming the hard (think water here), the rounded overcoming the straight (force) and the threaded overcoming the broken (force). It means that when a hard force (Gan) strikes out, the 'softer' rotational and diverting force (Rou) will redirect that straight and hard force and empty it of power. It can be diverted away or emptied into yourself through absorption. In any case, that ability must be trained. In practice it means the opponent's force is dissolved or led to its extreme limit, so compromising his stability. Either he will attempt to recover his stability or he will fall in the direction of his committed force. Either of these circumstances puts the opponent at a disadvantage. That is the point of attack, or better, should be described as the attack. In Taiji boxing the defensive strategy is also the attack, since there is no energetic break in the transition from one state to the other in the sense that block, and *then* strike, is clearly defend, and *then* attack. Ironing out the point of change is the skill of internalised boxing. In practice, attack and defence appear and feel simultaneous. This skill of changeability is called Zhuan Hua.

This is a core idea of Taiji boxing strategy, but obviously it is much more complex in actuality, and significant skills have to be acquired to divert, dissolve or absorb an aggressive, directed force. It is enough to say here that the primary thrust of training is defensive, since it is believed that, once these skills are acquired, it also serves as attack. Striking or kicking are often considered less important and are generally only applied once the opponent is already unstable. Attacking the joints, including the spine, is preferred to striking and kicking. The highest skills of Taiji are more in the realm of 'bouncing off' or 'throwing away', which means to project an opponent away from you with the minimum of effort. This is achieved through the medium of the attacker's own intention and force manipulated by a range of skills particular to Taijiquan. At the highest level, these skills are imperceptible to an observer, or indeed the attacker. Referred to as 'touch and fly' it is primarily these skills that have added to the mystique of Taijiquan as a boxing art and placed it on the top few rungs of the martial ladder.

Do not resist, do not let go

In terms of Yin and Yang the solo practice teaches us to feel the changes from substantial (solid) to insubstantial (empty) and to feel and control the degrees of transition, as well as learn and be comfortable with a physical vocabulary. When an opponent is involved, as in two-person training (Tui Shou), and force is directed at you, you must become 'empty' (Yin), at the point where he has projected his solid (Yang) force. This state is achieved by offering no resistance to an applied force; instead, yield and 'listen' to it (read as force and direction) and lead it to change. Typically, rotational movement is used to do this, and this rotation may be in the wrist, forearm, shoulder or waist, letting a 'folding' rotational sequence divert and dissolve incoming force. This is not the same as blocking, which is force against force.

Typically, on feeling the application of a force, you might react by tensing up or moving away as quickly as you can. Tension, of course, is resistance, which means the opponent's force can impact upon something 'substantial' and thus affect your ability to respond, and/or your stability. Moving away too quickly means you may lose contact with the force, providing a gap for further attack. Both responses have to be modified through training so that you do not meet an attack with resistance and you move only in accordance with the speed, force and direction of the attack, critically trying to keep in contact with it. This way you study the method of 'listening' (Ting Jin) and then interpreting (Dong Jin) the attacking force, or you may lose your ability to 'read' it. A student who has begun the training for these skills may typically become too 'loose' (i.e. no structure), thereby allowing the force to turn or dominate him too much, accelerating him into an unfavourable position. Keeping your centre and hence the dynamic integrity of the body is extremely important. Too loose, and loss of dynamic integrity and balanced and rooted movement compromises your martial ability and, in a real struggle, would mean defeat.

The saying 'do not resisit and do not let go' (Bu Diu, Bu Ding) expresses the two characteristics that are defining principles in the fighting strategy of Taijiquan. 'Resistance' means to use force to meet force, and 'not letting go' means to maintain a structure and internal tension so that the body is responsive to the force (without resistance) and can remain attached to it and move in accordance with it, without compromising your own stability. For the attacker, not finding resistance in the intended target causes both instability and a reflex to recover stability, unless committed beyond recovery, and this provides opportunity for the defender to attack.

The idea of keeping in contact with the attacking force while allowing its unhindered passage allows you to guide it away from your centre and, by applying a rotational force, accelerate and lead it to a point where its power is dissipated, causing the opponent either to stumble or to attempt a recovery. In addition, staying in contact means that you can interpret that force, its strength and direction, and simultaneously make contact with the centre of the issuing force.

This is a complex skill and requires considerable training. It is the key area of contact training that is undertaken in Taijiquan. It is not just a case of being relaxed. This is only the first hurdle. It requires a high level of subtle and integrated force as well as 'listening' and 'interpreting' skills. The touch skills required to achieve this are centred on the ideas of adhesion (Zhan), 'sticking to like glue' (Nian), 'linking with' (Lian) and 'following' (Sui), and along with 'do not resist and do not let go', comprise the core of Taiji martial strategy. All two-man practice is designed to develop these skills.

Foundation skills

In Taiji the process begins with the study of five defining skills which are the prerequisite of all further Taiji boxing development. Without them the martial ability will remain in the realms of 'push and shove', and although you might excel at this, it will not be Taijiquan. They are 'adhere to' (or 'connect with'), 'stick to', 'join with', 'follow' and 'don't resist and don't let go'.

'Adhere' is the skill of intercepting an attacking limb and making contact with it. (Body contact also requires these skills.) It is generally referred to the use of the arms and hands to achieve contact with the nearest or most appropriate part of the attacker's force, commonly the forearm or the elbow of an attacking fist. It may be on the outside of the arm or on the inside, on top or rising from below to achieve adhesion. Like a wet or moist hand, once the hand makes contact it seems to adhere to the surface. To achieve this, the hand is relaxed and 'full' but light and inquiring. The need for the defender to make contact with the aggressive force is the critical beginning of a sequence of rapid actions that are designed to listen and interpret, then redirect or dissolve the force and the direction of the opponent's attack.

'Sticking to' comes next in this four-phase process. To 'stick to' implies the idea of being glued. Indeed, the Chinese word Nian means 'glutinous', like sticky rice. Imagine a grain of rice stuck to your hand. It is hard to shake off. The quality of its stickiness is persistent and light.

The initial adhesion becomes 'glued' (stuck) to the surface at the point of first contact. Not just surface-to-surface like paper to paper, but a deeper sticking that binds the point of contact together and allows the defender to 'grasp' the deeper tissue of the point of contact. This is done not by grabbing, but by a slight, unobtrusive pressure. This then becomes the 'link' or 'joining with'.

The 'joining with' implies that awareness at the point of contact becomes deeper, as if penetrating the surface. 'Linking with' means to connect with the tissue and muscle beneath the surface and read the force. It is both subtle and quick, but to achieve it means to give up your own intention, to become empty (Yin) and perceptive to the opponent through touch. His Yang to your Yin, his hardness to your softness – from this comes the idea of 'joining' or 'linking with' not just the limb but the opponent's centre, intention and energetic quality. At this point you may sense the fulcral point of the attack.

'To follow' comes last in the four-phase skill that is the defining method of Taijiquan martial strategy. 'To follow' means not to impede your opponent's force but, having adhered, stuck to, connected with it, your entire body and footwork and rotational skills must work to accomodate the attack. The force of the attack can either be dissolved by allowing it to expend itself in its original direction, diverted away from you and manipulated over the period of its trajectory, or folded back to the opponent. The essential idea is to use your connection with the opponent to exploit his balance and his irreversibly committed force.

In the beginning it is, first, not easy to be calm and relaxed in the face of an attack. Second, to be really effective it is necessary to intercept the primary thrust of the attack; and third, 'listening' and interpreting that attack determines the appropriate response. The ability to listen and interpret are born out of the four-phase practice of adhere, stick, join and follow, which begins with the practice of 'pushing hands' (Tui Shou). This sequence is the fundamental skill, and along with 'don't resist and don't let go', comprises the basic mental and physical training both to overcome reflex tensions and to train the subtlety and control of the response. Training means continually refining these strategies and methods to a single movement that is both precise and capable of changing at any point.

Changeability is also a defining characteristic of the internal boxing arts, and generally the hard, Yang aspect is held back and hidden in the soft, rotational movements of the defender. It is released only when the opponent's centre is compromised and his Energy confused. This allows the defender to accommodate and change with the attacker in any phase of the engagement. In reality the attack must be dealt with quickly, and advanced skills mean the ability to blend defence and attack into one clear and succinct movement. Defence and attack are simultaneous, though defence skills must be acquired before attack skills emerge, in the same way as Yin characteristics are cultivated first and the Yang is nurtured and cultivated slowly.

Pushing hands

The foundation for all the fighting skills of Taijiquan are trained through the two-man exercises commonly referred to as 'pushing hands' (Tui Shou). Pushing hands is a system of learning both the foundational skills and later martial application, prior to free-style sparring.

It begins with single-hand operations and progresses to complex rotational and circular movements of large circle and later small circle pushing hands. To begin with the two partners face each other and alternate between the forward archery stance (Gong Bu) and the sit back posture (Xu Bu), maintaining contact at first with one hand, and then with both hands. That contact is through the back of the hand/wrist, and then the back of the hand/wrist and the elbow. Typically both partners use a rotational, horizontal 'milling' action or a more complex exchange that follows both horizontal and vertical, or at least a diagonally oriented circular rotation. Within this practice the core manipulations that are the eight methods, or energies, of Taijiquan are studied and perfected.

In addition to the hand manipulations, advanced practice teaches foot strategies for stepping across and around your opponent, as well as following and retreating. These are the 'five doors' and are extremely important boxing skills. Without the footwork, the hand manipulations are not enough.

Pushing hands can become very refined. The main aim is to study how to compromise and exploit your opponent's balance within movement and to maintain your own equilibrium in both defence and attack. Martial advantage is the result of exploiting the dynamics of the opponent's balance by using deception and lever-age either to attack the joints or vulnerable points on the body, or to throw the opponent away when his root has been severed and his ability to orientate himself towards you is confused. Pushing hands can be likened to a dialogue of questions and answers. My opponent pushes me, I divert, and immediately return an attack; he immediately senses it and prepares to defend; I change and my attack disappears; he immediately prepares to take advantage – and so it goes on. The better your opponent, the more complex the 'dia-logue' becomes. Beyond being martial training it is also enormously enjoyable.

The system of 'sticking or pushing' hands is not confined to Taijiquan but is also used in other martial systems to study attack and defence techniques. However, it is a signature practice in Taiji boxing training and has evolved into a very comprehensive method from which all the basic and advanced skills of Taiji boxing can be trained. In China, pushing hands has become an aspect of Taiji training that is an end skill in itself, and the defining skill that proves one's Taiji ability. However, pushing hands skill alone does not necessarily mean that you are a good fighter, since boxing ability is more complex than technical ability alone.

From fixed-step and moving-step pushing hands, it is also possible to train the methods of martial application (Yong Fa). Applications are the martial potential of the forms and movement that comprise the Taijiquan slow and fast forms, etc. Application of the movements combines both defence and attack aspects of Taiji and teaches you how to turn your defence into attack. There are many variations, but at the heart of Taiji boxing strategy is the anomaly that martial response is always determined by the movement of the attacker and as such cannot be predicted. The logical outcome of Taiji boxing is quite 'abstract' in that its action is always determined by the action of another. There should be no need for a drilled, pre-set response, and in fact such training might be considered counter-productive.

In Essence this means that whatever the opponent tries to do, whether strike or grapple, his attempts are futile, since his intention and his actions are diffused either at their inception or along the path, or even on arrival. The attacker in effect hurts himself when the defender separates the attacker's intention from his martial power, providing the gap that produces the most effective entrance for attack with an apparent minimum of effort (minimum effort to maximum effect). This is the level that is most highly regarded in China, since it appears both mysterious and to defy normal physics.

Pushing hands is both fulfilling and fascinating and can be practised even by those who have no interest whatsoever in martial arts. It is often said that the solo forms develop the martial vocabulary, the energetic and the physical body and mental skills, whereas the two-man exercises of pushing hands further develop the skills of balance, exchange and the understanding of Yin and Yang (as well as developing martial skills). There is no doubt that even for those with no interest in martial arts, the practice of pushing hands enhances their understanding of the solo forms.

In addition, pushing hands builds personal courage and confidence in interpreting other people's intentions and physical presence.

Practising in close physical contact with others over a long period allows you to address many issues regarding your own psychological and physical comfort zones. This is in itself a significant achievement, and one that many timid or anxious people can benefit from. Conversely, those over-confident and more bullish, achievement-oriented personalities who gravitate to dominance can learn much about moderation and gaining achievement from a different perspective.

The practice of pushing hands is built upon the platform of co-operation where two people come together to develop certain skills. The process reveals aspects of yourself which you may not be in touch with. This could be anything from fear to aversion, to anger and aggression to resistance. Remember that Taiji exploits the dynamics of balance in both yourself and another, and balance is both a physical and a mental state. When it is compromised, more rises to the surface than just the fear of falling. In this way Taiji pushing hands can also have a therapeutic function besides its original martial purpose.

Eight gates and five doors

The principle of 'use the least effort to produce maximum results' is the key to understanding the boxing strategy of Taijiquan. In fact it also serves as an excellent strategy for many aspects of our daily life.

In the martial application, the defender is constantly seeking an advantage by trying to drain his opponent's force, exploit the dynamics of his balance and use leverage and rotation to create advantage. Key to this is the ability to listen to and interpret your opponent, and for this contact is necessary. Contact always employs the four phases of 'sticking Energy', for without this there is no Taijiquan. It is the key Yin skill. Once this has been achieved and the opponent is disadvantaged, then the Yang aspect of attack can be expressed.

The blending and seamless change from defence to attack (Zhuan Hua), from Yin to Yang, is a refined skill and may take a long time to develop. In advanced practitioners this exchange can be immediate.

This skill is supplemented and infused with eight patterns of skills that are referred to as Eight Gates (Ba Men) or Eight Energies (Ba Jin), and these are the 'hardware' of Taiji boxing vocabulary (see below). They generally refer to hand manipulations but do in fact include body movement as methods of attack and defence. Energy is expressed in different ways, giving rise to a multitude of martial applications.

Energy is referred to as Jin and has special connotations in Taijiquan. It is a trained Energy and is the result of integrated movement, sinking/rooting, forward and backward changes and rotational Energy, combined with an elastic ability to compress and store Energy within the structure of the body and release it at will.

Releasing Energy is referred to as Fa Jin, or emitting 'trained power' or 'intrinsic Energy'. It is worth mentioning here that the word Jin describes the kind of Energy that is cultivated in the internal martial arts. It is not the Energy that is associated with muscle power and described as strength. It would be wrong to imply that the power of the muscles is not part of Jin, but Jin is actually more than this. It is the power that is developed by stretching, softening and dissolving blockages in the muscles, ligaments and tendons, as well as the overall connective tissue structure of the internal landscape. This allows for pathways of unhindered energetic flow to be cultivated for martial usage through specific movement practice. Jin is the rooted ground force transmitted, unhindered, through the body.

The Eight Gates are: Peng, Lu, Ji, An, Cai, Lie, Zhou and Kao. All the Eight Gates assume that the four-phase skill of sticking Energy (Zhan Nian Jin) and the principle of 'do not resist and do not let go' (Bu Dui, Bu Ding) have been understood, though in reality the two primary energies of Peng (Yang) and Lu (Yin) are studied simultaneously in the early exercises practice of Tui Shou, and are inseparable from the four phases and the governing rule of martial contact.

Of the eight, Peng is the primary energetic skill and all the other energies are built upon this. Peng is the buoyant Energy that supports an incoming force. It is the Energy that is 'adhere and stick to', 'join with and follow'. It is an Energy that receives the information regarding the nature of the force. It is the result of the body's ability to absorb force throughout its connective tissue and compress internally downward, while at the same time expanding outward to 'buoy up' and raise, or expand towards or beyond, the fulcrum of a force. Peng Jin is a stored energetic potential and the foundation Energy. It is therefore an integral part of all other seven energetic modes.

Developing Peng is one of the great difficulties in Taijiquan, since without it there can be no knowledge of the other gates. Peng is the primary martial Energy and is the result of consistent and prolonged form practice and the practice of pushing hands. It is the best reason to practise the two-man exercises, since they are important in the development and refinement of Peng Jin. Think of the solo practice as having one sealed end, which is the ground, against which the body pushes to create the counterforce necessary to our functional relationship with the world around us. The other end is our hands. Martial activity must teach us to receive Energy inwards and either divert, dissolve or dissipate it. But the connection to an incoming force at the top end (hands, arms, etc.) and the upward pushing force of the ground end must reconcile itself throughout the whole system. Within the closed system that is created by the body, between the point of received force and the ground, there must be a reconciliation, a storing and a return. Peng Jin is this reconciliation of forces and the held potential of return. It is not associated with muscle tension, and is considered to be developed first in the legs. Through practice and awareness it then migrates upwards, eventually filling out the whole structure. It is a strongly felt sensation.

Training Peng is done through form practice, at first from cultivating the empty and substantial quality in the legs and the forward and backward exchange of full and empty and, also important, is the transition of weight loading. In the early stages it will not be possible to feel a commensurate sensation in the arms, since they have no ground to push against, but the skill of understanding substantial and insubstantial in the arms and how the transition from one to the other works, and then how they are informed by the same in the legs is the result of pushing hands, partner experience where tangible sensations are commited to body memory, and then the solo form practice. Pushing hands practice makes the solo form feel, and indeed look, different than if you do not undertake this important aspect of training.

The baseline for developing Peng Energy must be the state of relaxed alignment (Song Jin) and the consequent correct shape, creating a dynamic that is balanced, co-ordinated, mobile and able to transmit and move internal Energy and received Energy efficiently. 'Pole standing' and forms of dynamic Qi Gong are also typical methods of cultivating Peng Energy in the legs and translating that quality of Energy into the upper body and then the arms.

From Peng Energy comes Lu Energy, which is a Yin-associated Energy. It is concerned with diverting and is generally referred to as a 'rolling back' Energy. Lu is a quality of movement that is built on Peng as its foundation. It is typified by the body's rotational ability, employed during the four phases of attaching. Rotational skills start with, and are all governed by, the waist (pelvis), but later more sophisticated rotations of the forearm and hands are developed. Additional forwards or pulling-back movements of the arms can be combined with clockwise or anti-clockwise rising or falling rotations of the arms, connected to the rotation of the waist and forwards and backwards movement of the legs. Together, an incredible, light but effective and complex integrated force can be achieved that is used to fully divert an incoming force away from your centre to either partially dissipate or fully divert the force accordingly. The degree and direction of circularity, of course, is determined by the appropriate response to the incoming force. Understanding this skill depends upon two-man exercises where the need to reconcile forces that are aimed at destabilising you is real. The degree of turn and angle of arc, etc., are all learned in pushing hands and then refined endlessly until they are seamless and almost invisible to the casual observer.

Although Lu is a Yin Energy, combining yielding and softness, it is not without the expansive and buoyant structure that comes from Peng. Without this, Lu would easily collapse and lose its martial ability. Refinement of Lu results from understanding the amount of rotation and the effectiveness and degree of the arcs that comprise the overt aspects of the 'rolling back'. Peng and Lu are fundamental energetic qualities, without which Taiji skills cannot be developed.

From Peng and Lu, Ji and An are developed. Ji is a straight force and is the primary attacking force of Taiji boxing. It is associated with a punch, kick, or most commonly with a 'press', where the back of one hand is placed against an opponent. On completion of inward rolling movement the other hand is placed, palm out, against the hand or wrist and, combined with the forward momentum from the pushing leg, projects Energy through the hands into the opponent. It is also a rebounding force that shoots out as soon as the opponent's force has been diverted or neutralised. Ji can come from any part of the body and it is as if the Energy on landing is repelled in the same direction or line of attack. It can also be applied from any direction, aimed at the opponent's centre line.

In Taiji boxing strategy, a striking hand or foot is often placed upon the opponent before the Energy is released. It can effect a drilling or deeply penetrating and explosive force, or a softer, disruptive and disabling attack aimed at dislodging the opponent's centre, attacking a joint or an acupressure point. You should already be in contact with the opponent and their balance should already be disrupted if you are to 'shoot' or 'press' Energy into them. A high-level practitioner, once having made contact, would effect disruption of balance very quickly and apply Ji Jin simultaneously.

An Jin (pushing Energy) is both a defensive and an attacking method. It is considered a smothering and downward tending force, and is associated with the power and effects of water. It is able to subdue and calm attacking force and exhibit enormous pushing power, accelerating evenly into the opponent and pressing their centre downward and also away, thereby facilitating a return rising force within the opponent as they attempt to recover from the downward pressure. This is sometimes seen as an opponent bouncing upwards and away in their attempt to recover their stability, or else being pushed into the ground. Typically, the double-handed push in Taiji is the signature gesture most commonly referred to as An.

These four constitute the main strategic and energetic skills of Taijiquan and they appear in various combinations in all of the martial vocabulary. The next four strategic martial energies (Jin) are Pull Down (Cai), Split (Lie), Elbow\forearm stroke (Zhou) and Bumping or shoulder stroke (Kao).

Cai is associated with a plucking action, as if pulling something downwards. Its primary expression is known as 'needle at sea bottom' where the diverting/roll back is transformed into a rapid downward, pulling action, shocking the opponent and raising their centre and impacting upon their shoulder joint and neck. Done more discreetly, it is a common strategy to 'pluck' the opponent's force forward and downwards to topple them or compromise their balance. It has many uses and is an important energetic skill.

Lie is associated with splitting something or separating it from its source. The action of Lie is generated by rotation of the waist and the stretching out and separating ability of the arms in contact with the opponent. Your hands can move either in opposite directions, thereby stretching your opponent in two directions, or in the same direction in a downward arc that separates the opponent from his root. Generally the action of Lie requires an oblique angle in relation to your opponent, giving you rotational advantage or opening a slight gap for one hand, to penetrate to the body as the other draws the opponent's hand and arm out against the will of the joint.

Zhou or what is commonly called 'elbow stroke' actually refers to the elbow and the forearm. It can be a powerful 'stab' with the elbow point, or a pounding force of the forearm, or a rotational force that folds across the opponent's incoming strike (particularly the arm) and folds up his elbow, thereby throwing him off balance. It is a lock that is both powerful and immediate. It is the integrated rotational force of the waist and shoulder, transmitted to the rotational arc of the elbow, that empowers the forearm. Zhou is associated with this 'folding' ability of the arm to collapse through its joint to both dissipate force and seek advantage. As it collapses primarily through the elbow, an arc of return is sensed. The folding inward process can then be folded back out against your opponent.

Kao or 'shoulder stroke' (sometimes referred to as 'leaning' or 'bumping') in its simplest form is an attack with the shoulder to the opponent's midline. It can be employed at very close range. However, such an attack can also be released from any part of the torso, the back being particularly powerful. Critically in this form of attack the Taiji player must have good control of his centre and judge the distance well. It is common to incline too much and thereby compromise your balance. The power is a fully integrated force driven by the legs, but it can also be applied by a rapid rotation, causing the whole torso to rotate quickly and release force. This is a more unusual variation, as is simply walking into your opponent and bumping him violently with your upper torso to project him backwards. The more common shoulder stroke is also associated with the idea of folding Energy, since an opponent's force, when folded up, often ends up at the player's shoulder, as if they have fallen onto it. 'Folding' is either defence or attack, or simultaneously both, and each part (fingers, palm, wrist, forearm, elbow and shoulder) can be trained to strike and to facilitate locking up and dissipating an opponent's force.

In Taiji these movements are considered as particular expressions of internal Energy and must be trained. Their training is done primarily in pushing hands, which allows many combinations of movement while training the 'adhere/stick/connect and follow' strategy and the very difficult and extraordinary skill of non-resistance. They appear in different combinations and may alternate rapidly from one to the other.

In Taiji boxing training, as in all martial arts, the ability to move intelligently, strategically and swiftly from one place to another is clearly important. In Taiji language this is basically defined as 'advance, retreat, step to the left to attack right, go to the right to attack left' and what is referred to as 'central equilibrium', which denotes the stability of all movement, as well as referring to turning. It is a state of continual balance and is present in the other steps, just as Peng Jin must be in all the eight methods, as previously discussed.

The aim of the Taiji footwork is to be responsive in 'following' the opponent's direction of force, as well as to be able to step around the opponent's line of force to attack the side or back, or any angle that is appropriate to the attacker's movement. Achieving the hand skills means that the opponent's force can be detected, diverted or controlled and his martial intention interpreted. To thwart his martial intention means to take up a favourable position that provides access to his vulnerable areas. It is sometimes said that boxing skills are 70 per cent footwork.

Circles and straight lines, gathering and releasing

In advanced practice, defence and attack become virtually simultaneous and the different defensive and attacking phases combine and blend in a continuous and seamless exchange between the soft defensive (Yin) and hard attacking (Yang) phases. Often alternating rapidly to disorientate the opponent and seek the most advantageous moment, the ability to transfer from one state into another (Zhuan Hua) is a high-level skill. It takes a long time to develop these skills, and a lot of patience, which is possibly why few Taiji practitioners reach a high level and so many fall off the long ladder.

There are particular characteristics that allow movement to alternate between soft (Rou) and hard (Gan) Energy. The first is the characteristic of 'roundness'. It guides and defines the general shape and appearance of Taiji movement and is essentially expressed in the Yin aspect of Taiji boxing. 'Soft' does not mean that the physical structure becomes floppy and collapsible, but that within the constraints of the structure the 'rounded' shapes are preferable. The rounded shape adds connectivity and determines optimum angles of the joints that permit the easy transfer of Energy from the ground up and the hands down. Roundness allows for fluidity in movement, storage of energetic potential, change and continuity. Roundedness is an expression of Peng Energy.

On a simple level, the body must be like an inflated ball. The ball rotates to repel an applied force as well as partially or wholly absorb it (as a softly inflated ball can). Both aspects are important to diverting, yielding and absorbing the opponent's force. Imagine a ball full of Energy (Qi), equal in pressure throughout and able to 'soak' up force across the whole interior, as well as divert it by rotating to throw it off. There are degrees of rotation and absorption and they are dependent on the force and direction of the opponent. A common error in studying this aspect of Taiji is to overexpress the rotation needed to divert a force, leading to an excess within your own posture and thence a weakness.

In Taiji the body (spine) and limbs are considered to be like bows that must bend to absorb and store Energy, and lengthen or straighten to express or issue Energy. The bow in its most potent status is bent, but if bent too far the potential is released by the bow snapping. Taiji is the same: too much curve or too little curve are both failings. In solo practice the optimum curvature must be achieved for comfort, energetic integrity, continuity and change. In pushing hand practice the optimum curve must be refined to divert and dissolve force applied against you in a multitude of angles and intensity. Stability and a loose rotational ability within the joints is the key. Any resistance will allow a straight line force to find a point of entry to your centre. Non-resistance plus rotational skills and a curved surface make it more difficult for a force to impact upon your stability or find adequate purchase to shut you down.

The circular nature of Taiji movement is made possible by the rotational ability of the waist and the curving ability of the spine and its relationship to the rotational ability of the shoulders, elbows, wrists and hands. In motion, the curves are led by the hands and power rises up and down as required. Large circular movements are easily generated by the rotational ability of the waist, and this is one of the early stage skills that are developed in solo work, but contact with another force, as in pushing hands, means we must develop extending and expanding movements and inward and contracting movement. This is achieved by rotational and spiralling skills that augment the grosser rotations of the pelvis. The clockwise and counter-clockwise movements that are expressed in the arms and hands augment the movement of the waist and spine. The movement is led by the hands and, combined with the rotational ability of the forearms, is a powerful penetrating, drilling and disrupting force, as well as a diverting and guiding force. By cultivating all the rotational and circular capabilities of the body and integrating them in movement you can achieve a high level of refinement and integrated force. That force, when expressed in a circular way, can be both continuous and soft, while simultaneously storing Energy.

At any point in the continuously curving and rotating movements that are Taiji you must be able to express that Energy in the manner of a damaging attack. This means releasing a significant amount of Energy into the opponent (Fa Jin) in a way that is unexpected, disruptive and instantaneous.

We have already discussed the creation of opportunity, and when the gap opens, the continuous curving movements of defence must direct an energetic release at the opponent. This skill is difficult to achieve and must be trained. The soft and circular must, in a split second, become hard and directed (straight). From the arcing spiral or rotation of the body the stored Energy must be projected from a single point into the opponent. This process is called 'turning the circle into the square' and denotes the attacking phase of Taiji engagement.

This is one of the most important skills in Taiji boxing if it is ever to become fully useful as a martial art. It is the result of long practice, cultivating the 'Taiji body' and developing sophisticated control of the body. Your attack is an energetic burst radiating from your centre and releasing Energy into, or through, a single point of contact. With practice it can be released from almost any part of your body, but typically from hand, forearm and elbow, legs, shoulder and back. It can only be achieved if the body is relaxed in a way that stores energetic potential and at the same time is totally responsive to directed intention to allow that potential to be released. This is the ability to transform from soft (Yin) and circular to hard (Yang) and directed in a split second. To take it further you must be able to return just as quickly to that state of soft roundness.

Gathering and releasing – water, the bow and the whip

The most common analogy for understanding the energetic and physical qualities that we try to cultivate in Taiji, and indeed all Qi Gong, is water. The cleansing, nourishing, permeating and revitalising aspects of water readily translate as the free movement and balanced distribution of Energy (Qi) that is the aim of Qi Gong. It also represents the continually changing state that is our living experience and is represented in the theory of Yin–Yang.

In the martial terms of internal boxing it is the soft, liquid, yielding and penetrating nature of water that conceals the hard destructive potential (Yang within Yin). In Taiji as in Qi Gong, the body must be transformed into a flexible and integrated whole that exhibits the fluidity of water in movement. In stillness, muddy water clears and this represents the quiescent state of mind. The idea of blood and Qi reaching every last cell of the body is that of a body gently irrigated, nourished and cleansed in the way water irrigates crops and, when propelled, flushes out blocked and silted canals.

In a martial analogy Qi, like water, fills out and supports all the functioning of the body, and the martial forces referred to as Jin are like powerful currents. Those currents are generated by shaped movement, contact and absorption, storage, and the steady pressure of internal, downward tidal forces rebounding off the ground like waves off a sea wall. It is the creation, cultivation, harnessing and directing of this force that concerns the Taiji martial player.

In the Taiji community the body is considered to have five bows (as in bow and arrow). These bows are the arms, legs and spine, and are the primary means of storing and releasing Energy, as well as transforming it into martial power. The bows are mutually supportive and maintain an optimum curve, both vertically and (in the case of the arms) horizontally. In the receiving phases of defence, where absorption and dissipation of a force is most needed, the bones, muscles, ligaments, tendons and connective tissue all work together to compress, store and dissolve the opponent's Energy. In the attack phase that Energy is released through a particular point (hand, fingers, foot, etc.) by the lengthening of the bows and the release of stored Energy like an arrow, throughout the body.

The release of Energy can be fast and penetrating, like an arrow, or slow, powerful and deep, like the pounding or surging action of a wave, or accelerating like the wave action of a whip. The analogy of the whip serves to describe the wavelike action of Energy as it is generated in the feet and legs (the whip handle), accelerating and controlled by the rotation of the waist, released up along the spine and chanelled to a hand, as if from the handle to the tip of the whip, in a continuous wave that is released at the end, undiminished. With little apparent loss of Energy from source to release, Energy is magnified and directed in a single, continuous thread.

In defence, and once contact is made, the four phases of contact must ensue and the strategy of 'don't resist and don't let go' must be adhered to. Energy from the opponent is diverted and/or absorbed. Absorption dissolves Energy into the ground through the feet but also stores it within and across the whole internal structure. Externally this generally appears as a compacting, sinking and pulling inwards movement called 'gathering'. Gathering is a defensive strategy. The other side of gathering is releasing, which is of course the attacking action where the absorbed Energy can be controlled and released in a specific direction. The physical action and the corresponding internal sensations are very particular, and the more practised, the more full and thoroughly connected they feel. By this I mean that the feet (on the ground) and the hands (on the opponent) are linked and the body sensation is harmonious, integrated and evenly full throughout (not just, for instance, in the hands).

As experience develops it becomes possible to discern and adjust the need for absorption and gathering in precise accordance with your opponent's force, as well as how much Energy to release, and in what direction. The apparent gathering and releasing becomes less obvious, until both inwards gathering and outwards releasing movement become almost simultaneous. This is a skill that must be studied through long practice of two-person manipulations (Tui Shou). Although it is hard to achieve the same sensations of fullness and functionality without pushing hands, it is still possible in the solo forms to achieve a feeling of gathering the potential Energy generated by dynamic movement and study the mechanism whereby the whole body can store Energy in compression and release it to a particular point by lengthening.

Fighting, fun, weapons and the point

Since Taijiquan is a martial art it should, by definition, serve that end. However, its modern development has clearly created a split between practice for recreation and health and the practice for martial proficiency. Indeed, the methods of practice also diverge within the martial route.

It has become quite common practice in China and in the West for the health practice to precede the martial knowledge, and in many cases for the martial knowledge, and practice to be completely ignored. This is a pity, since the vocabulary, methods and strategies of Taiji boxing are fascinating. In addition, they change the value of the solo forms, giving them substance by reinforcing and articulating the physical and the energetic components. However there are degrees of the martial, and many people settle for the solo form and a little pushing hands. Indeed, pushing hands has become a highly respected art in itself, since it can both exercise basic martial skills and provide a forum for studying the subtle skills of Taijiquan.

However it must be said that pushing hands alone cannot produce a fighter, though without first achieving pushing hands skills the fighter would not be practising Taiji boxing. Pushing hands is a bridge that must be crossed successfully before Taijiquan can become martial.

You cannot easily ignore the martial nature of Taijiquan, since it is very evident in its mechanics, postures, and so on. Their profundity and effectiveness are best explored by investigating the boxing skills, methods and strategies. Basic martial skills firm up integrated and precise movement, as well as refining the postural requirements, balance and ability to exploit the dynamics of balance in oneself and one's opponent. In addition there are other benefits, such as increased mental and physical confidence, courage, and the kind of mental focus and skills that Taiji boxing trains.

In addition to martial skills that build on the hand forms and pushing hands, there are also weapons forms. Before the advent of the gun all martial arts systems in China would have aimed to develop certain weapons. The most common weapons of Taijiquan are generally the double-edged sword, the broadsword, the spear (long and short) and pole.

The point of learning to use these mediaeval weapons is to develop and refine a more complex vocabulary of movements than the hand form, and to learn the different qualities of Energy that are required to use them. Each weapon lends something new and builds a greater skill base with enhanced versatility, as well as a more robust and capable co-ordinative mobility and strength.

The double-edged sword (Jian) is refined and accurate in its rotating and spiralling movements and its use of both edges and different cutting techniques. It develops wrist flexibility and connected rotational skills and requires you to integrate the body and sword in a light, responsive and energetic harmony from the foot to the tip of the sword. Physically, it demands stretching, long and deep stances, high stances and low twisted stances, single leg stances, jumps and kicks. In character it is the closest of all the weapons forms to the empty-hand form, though it is both more demanding and more complex. The double-edged sword is a sophisticated light weapon requiring great dexterity, skill and balance. It is beautiful both to do and to watch, having much in common with the art of calligraphy. It is considered to be the weapon of the educated and virtuous.

The broadsword (Dao) is the all-purpose weapon. It is heavier than the Jian and much more robust, without the responsive flexibility of the double-edged sword. Typically, the sharp edge is swept in large continuous arcs, interspersed with chops, stabs, hacking attacks and defensive blocks and divertions, while the blunt edge is often reinforced by the free hand, adding significant power and capability to it in close fighting. It is a powerful weapon and well suited to the battlefield. It builds strength and power in the upper body and deeply rooted stances. While the double-edged sword uses fine circles and flicking, drawing and sawing action from the wrist with light movement, the broadsword develops the back, rotational power generated in the legs, control in the waist, strength and endurance.

The spear (Qiang) and the pole (Gan) are difficult weapons owing to their length and the need to use both ends and both hands simultaneously. The large circles generated by the spear and pole increase your reach in defence and attack and this requires a special control over the fulcrum, the two hands and the ends of the weapon. Indeed, the fulcrum of the spear or pole must link to your own centre if the constant rotations and exchanges are to have connectivity, sensitivity and power. These two weapons are demanding on the shoulders, arms and lower back, and the spear puts additional stress on the upper body and structural integrity of the postures, owing to its length and the large, sweeping and circular movements. The use of both right and left hands in a constant energetic exchange allows you to develop the left side more thoroughly. Power is shared equally by alternating pulling and pushing and taking advantage of the weight of the weapon. It also develops the rotational skill of the wrist and the power of the waist.

The skill and achievement of wielding the spear (and one of the reasons why it is considered the king of all the weapons) is in cultivating perfect manipulative and striking control at a distance from your centre. Its vocabulary combines both the sweeping, arcing actions of the broadsword and the accurate smaller rotations and piercing skills of the double-edged sword.

Skills fostered in pushing hands are further developed by the practice of the double-edged sword, spear and pole. 'Sticking' weapons routines, which are an advanced form of weapons play similar to pushing hands, are a wonderful addition to a weapons syllabus, as are the duelling forms that exist in some Taiji systems.

There is no doubt that studying at least one weapon is advantageous to your development and appreciation of Taijiquan. It will also increase your physical integrated strength and muscle tone, balance and co-ordination. Typically that weapon might be the double-edged sword, since the core strategies and internal work required of Taiji hand techniques are most clearly applicable to and developed by using the double-edged sword. Its two-man 'sticking swords' practice is also closely related to pushing hands.

Taijiquan and the daily grind

As a martial art Taijiquan offers strategies that meet our everyday needs. The study of Taijiquan does not mean that you have to be personally disposed to fighting or confrontation. Neither does it mean that you need to be subject to a bruising regime of press-ups on one finger, or being regularly knocked about, bruised and abused, although for some this can be quite enjoyable and rewarding. Taijiquan stradles a martial and a health culture, and this may in the end be its real strength and relevance in our modern world. The martial can be tempered to promote health-giving qualities and health-seekers can learn something from the martial. Weapons form training is a good example of a practice that is physically demanding and elegant, even though you may never have a swordfight with anybody in your life. Taiji pushing hands is a practice that perfectly balances martial skills with enhanced understanding of the Taiji principles. In a co-operative relationship with your partner it can be physically and mentally rewarding, without necessarily involving the fear of being 'decked'.

Pushing hands is both the study of balance and dynamics and an interesting window onto your own nature, and indeed your partner's. Much is revealed when balance is questioned by way of physical manipulation and opposition, and being in close physical contact with another person, their mental state and their physicality can sometimes be very disconcerting. Indeed the whole process of learning the complex co-ordination of the hand manipulations in fixed and moving step sequence seems to affect us at a deep functional and psychological level, and it is to our benefit.

Following the Taiji boxing principle of meeting force with no resistance means giving up the deeply ingrained mechanism of resistance (meeting force with force). Learning to give this up is more than just a rewiring of our reflexes: it must be realised at the much deeper level of our innate nature. It is a relinquishing of our physical, and sometimes our emotional defences. The resulting vulnerability is the exposure of our 'centre' and all that that implies, in both physical and mental respects. In Taijiquan there is much talk about investing in loss. This means that only after relinquishing resistance can you truly achieve the skills of protecting your centre and exploiting the dynamics of your opponent's equilibrium. It is a remarkable idea and system and evolves progressively as you allow yourself to be exposed until you find the skills and the mentality to perceive, interpret and respond. Giving up resistance means not only physical resistance but emotional and intellectual resistance too.

Taijiquan is a formidable and highly respected martial art, so investing in loss does not mean 'loser'. It means that there comes a point of recognition where loss becomes gain and the principles and methods that make up the strategy of Taijiquan begin to emerge. Confidence grows in listening to, interpreting and responding to the prevailing conditions appropriately with the least resistance and effort. This is a defining characteristic of Taijiquan. It is the emergence of the 'Yang from Yin', that is movement from stillness, attack from defence and something from nothing. It is a state of mind as much as a martial skill and its benefits in daily life are enormous. You meet force and resistance all around, as well as the myriad agendas and intentions of others impinging on your own path and stability. Having a strategy rooted in the body knowledge of Taiji form practice and pushing hands helps us to negotiate this.

The idea of cultivating non-resistance as a personal and social strategy for surviving our daily circumstances does not mean that you are constantly walked over by those with stronger intentions and more aggression than you. It means that a lot of what might previously have led you into emotional or physical conflict can be dissolved. Equanimity can rule and a still centre can be maintained while all around may seem like madness. Staying centred and relaxed leads to clarity and understanding. The strategies and mindset of Taiji are beautifully relevant to emotional as well as physical conflict. In addition, the development of the physical skills in pushing hands builds a mental repertoire for dealing with emotional conflict. This is one of the beautiful and profound by-products of the study of Taijiquan.

Taijiquan is called a 'soft' art and an 'internal' art, but it is also a way of life. It is the circle rather than the square, the soft rather than the hard, and the gentle rather than the aggressive. It is a path for both physical and mental health. Quiet, calm and non-resistant is the way of self-cultivation, conservation (nourishing life Energy) and rejuvenation (Eternal Spring).

The study of Taiji martial strategies is not just confined to attack and defence: it offers some transferable skills useful for dealing with many of the physical and emotional hurdles that may confront us in our modern world. It is not the same as the boxing and kick-boxing workouts and the rest of the gym systems that have been developed for people who will never kick or box. Taijiquan is a real and dynamic skill of physical and mental balance and stability.

Physical and emotional stability confer confidence and courage as well as accumulating and conserving life's vital Energy, and maintaining good functional mobility, flexibility and balance. We are under daily stress from our environment and sometimes from people who might wish to harm us or casually dump their stress or frustration onto us. The systems of the body and mind have a close relationship with our environment that can lead us towards either nurture or dissipation. A discipline that teaches us to guard our Energy against the destructive and negative forces and nurture the beneficial and positive forces is a move in the right direction. This is the way of Qi Gong and Taijiquan.

Thresholds, hurdles and maturity

Both Taijiquan and Qi Gong are subtle arts and they become increasingly more so, the more you practise. This is as true for those who practise for health as it is for the martial artist. In the process of reaching those subtle levels there are many thresholds of physical competence and mental achievement to cross. Everyone has them, and recognising and crossing them is evidence of progress.

Most beginners are surprised at the learning curve necessary to achieve basic skills in Qi Gong, and more especially Taijiquan. For the uninitiated they look deceptively simple.

The most common and first threshold that most people reach is that of their physical capability. Not everyone is able to meet their own expectations of what they can achieve physically. It seems we are not all born equal when it comes to physical and co-ordinative skills. A lack of these skills can make you feel awkward and consequently frustrated. Solving this problem, though, is generally as simple as practising more with a clear idea about how to do this correctly.

For most of you progress will be reasonably comfortable, providing you practise, and practise correctly. It is also necessary to accept that lack of physical ability or co-ordination or difficulties of balance are all slow to rectify. Capability often emerges slowly, and emotional frustrations or difficulties may dissolve slowly. They must be worked through with vigilant attention and persistent and regular practice. When the body is trained and the attention turned inwards, many emotional and physical problems can be dissolved and those thresholds can be crossed.

A more complex and perhaps more difficult threshold is when you have some habitual postural issue or tension that you are unable to correct, or that has gone unnoticed for many years. Correcting postural problems can be a long and slow process, since you have become accustomed to the compensatory state of your body. Such conditions are widespread and may have a whole raft of contributive causes. If they are deeply rooted and reinforced by emotional investment they are very difficult to change. If, however, they are simply the result of poor postural awareness and practice then it is much easier. A good introduction to postural awareness and persistent correction in class will help, and will generally go a long way to establishing new postural habits.

More complex are the psychological problems that often become evident in the practice of Qi Gong. Qi Gong consistently throws up emotional issues and stray (but strong) feelings. It is its power to release deeply held emotions that gives it its therapeutic value. Qi Gong alone may not be able to dissolve deep emotions, but in conjunction with other therapies it can offer a route to healing, or modify both debilitating physical conditions and emotional scarring.

For physically debilitating conditions, Qi Gong can offer a respite from tensions and a chance to deal with pain and mobility problems. It may never be possible to remove these conditions, but practice can be adjusted to account for them and there is no reason why people with long-term or inherited physical difficulties cannot practise Qi Gong to their benefit. Tailoring Qi Gong to suit the student's condition is important, and the teacher must have a depth of knowledge that allows for this. Taijiquan, for instance, may not be a viable option, but the range of Qi Gong movements can be edited to ensure both the possibility of practice and the benefits.

Few people, if any, are trouble-free when they come to Qi Gong or Taijiquan. Indeed, many come because they have problems that they believe can be solved by these disciplines. Often they can, or at least to a degree.

One of the great hurdles is taking your practice into daily life. This means being motivated to practise on your own, out of a class, and also it means thinking about posture, respiration, calming the emotional mind and taking every opportunity to look inward and rest from the daily sensory and informational assault. Walking, standing and sitting are opportunities to use the principles of Qi Gong.

Another common threshold is that of achieving deep relaxation and the energetic quality associated with it. At first we can follow the postural rules as we start practice, but to keep to those rules at all times is difficult. The levels of relaxation are several, each one bringing a new release and a deeper sense of comfort. What you often think of as being relaxed is only the first level, which becomes progressively deeper and deeper as you train yourself. Deep and short-term tensions can be relieved by maintaining an awareness of ourselves and of where those tensions are arising. Tension can quickly drive our body into stress mode, and this significantly disrupts the internal climate. We can learn to monitor ourselves and constantly remind ourselves to relax and listen to ourselves carefully for signs of discomfort.

Each stage of 'giving up' represents a threshold, and as bigger thresholds are crossed they become increasingly more subtle. In the beginning learning a set of movements may seem easy, even focusing attention for a brief period may seems quite easy to some, but as you progress new and unexpected sensations and difficulties, both physical and mental, may arise. Dealing with those difficulties can be a lengthy process.

Two such instances are the full releasing of the diaphragm in natural abdominal breath, and stilling the internal dialogue or chatter that constantly distracts you from the focused awareness necessary to achieve the full benefits of Qi Gong. The achievement of relaxing the diaphragm and stilling the chatter, even momentarily, will provide the impetus to keep at it. Success is the result of long practice, but both of these problems are stubborn and the latter, the chatter of the mischievous mind, is certainly the most difficult of all.

During the practice of the Taiji form you may notice a change in respiration as inhalation and exhalation become longer and more satifactory. You may even notice the diaphragm change as it progressively relaxes. This will be related to a 'giving up' sensation in the abdomen, a wall of muscle that is generally held in and therefore restricts natural breath and the working of the diaphragm. Similarly, chest and rib tension will do the same and a slow releasing, an unsticking, often occurs over the duration of a form set or after lengthy practice. This is an important achievement and a major threshold to unlocking the body and the mind for advanced practice. You may also notice little thresholds where the diaphragm becomes 'unstuck', or internal conversation just dissolves into a clear awareness of your movement and breath. It is like the runner who feels the first wave of resistance but carries on through the second, and maybe third, wave until the rhythm is achieved and the muscles and mind have acclimatised and settled. Spread over years of practice the thresholds become less obvious and the ability to cross them easier. In maturity thresholds still arise, and dissolve in a natural way.

Thresholds are a normal part of the journey and should not be considered negatively, but you do need to work through them before new realisations and new awarenesses become tangible and fully incorporated. This generally happens with hindsight, and what seems obvious now was perhaps not even on your horizon at the time. This is typical. The practice of Taiji and Qi Gong reveals much about you to yourself, both physically and mentally, and having a reflective intelligence is useful in discerning lines of improvement and achievement and the emergence of different thresholds, both physical and emotional. Patience and perseverance are important here.

One of the biggest thresholds to cross is your own expectation. Many people have preconceived ideas about what to expect, and also restrictive ideas about what they are able to do. Lack of progress is sometimes linked to limiting expectation, and also to expectations that exceed your particular stage of development. Realistic expectations of what can be achieved are important, and it is worth remembering that those expectations will change as knowledge and maturity of practice evolve, but it is also important to allow practice to unfold naturally and one step at a time. In this way the thresholds rise up in an evolutionary order and are crossed more comfortably.

Improvements are often brought about by a competent teacher who is able not only to teach you the the form, correct shape and body alignment, but also how the body, respiration and mind work together. A good teacher can also spot issues that are likely to retard your development, and can often lead you through thresholds of experience and guide you to a maturity of practice.

Prolonged practice brings a new awareness of the form(s) and shapes, which in turn allows incremental adjustments that then alter the sensations of both the external (physical) self and and internal (energetic) self. Crucially, corrective awareness is the means by which it is possible to monitor yourself posturally, and investigative aware-ness is the means of discovering the sensations within. Adjustments to posture can radically change the sensations that accompany a move-ment – and postural correctness is not just a beginner's problem. It can plague people whose deep-seated postural habits cannot be shifted. Real effort has to be made to keep self-awareness and self-correction at the top of the agenda – until, that is, you get it right.

Getting it right eventually feels both natural and comfortable and is the result of working through all your physical diffi-culties until the body emerges that exhibits the unrestrained, unforced and relaxed mobility and the fluid elastic strength and firm balance that are the achievement of Qi Gong and Taijiquan.

Correcting excess or deficiency in posture and movement is un-doubtedly one of the hardest aspects of 'getting it right'. We are often blind to our deficiencies and see our excesses sometimes as strengths. Deficiencies are often the result of distracted and unfo-cused thinking, and of not taking care with the external physical relationships and the linking internal sensations, not finishing the movements completely, not expressing the optimum connectivity of curves, arcs, spirals and rotations in expanding and contracting, and not paying proper attention to the transitions from weighted to empty in the process of stepping. All of these are basic ideas that need to be revisited even by the adept. You are never so good that you can neglect the basics, and each practice session should always revisit aspects of basic practice.

Just as deficiency must be addressed, so must excess. Excess may show up as too much leaning, or over-inclined posture; it may be too much muscle force, or exaggerated movements. It may also be a mental excess where ego invests too much in the beauty, elegance or martial appearance and meaning of a movement. Moderation is necessary and the 'middle path' is the right way.

The middle path is extremely important in the cultivation of the right body and mind, as well as in the duration and methods of practice. In Qi Gong it is important to finish feeling good and en-ergised, not completely exhausted. This is definitely a sign of more maturity in practice and indicates that you have learned just how much is required to accumulate, mobilise and store your Energy.

This should also be applied to the Taiji boxing training. Overly physical or stressful workouts can leave you feeling depleted, and tension arising from over-training can become counter-productive. However, it must also be said that there is a relationship in all body and mind work between effort and returns, 'pain and gain' and what is sometimes described in China as 'eating bitter'. In other words, you have to put in the hard work to reach the achievements. The trick is spreading the work over a long period of time in a calm and persistent way, not driven by an unrealistic agenda or too high an expectation. In China this is done by working at it daily in the parks, year after year. In the West it is often done by meeting once or twice a week in the evenings. The traditional Chinese way is undoubtedly the best, but generally it does not suit our Western lifestyle.

In wondering how to get better at your practice, it is always worth remembering the primary purpose of Qi Gong. That is: to regulate the body, the breath and the mind for the benefit of your health and to promote vitality and well-being. This is the first base also in Taiji boxing training, and is a path of self-cultivation.

Self-cultivation means working on yourself, and the place to start is on your body. It is often a real eye-opener, and when people start to do Qi Gong or Taiji they often feel uncomfortable 'in themselves'. Indeed, their physical awkwardness is sometimes very obvious and clearly indicates a separation between mental and physical activity. Early stages of practice can be like putting a magnifying class to yourself and seeing aspects of yourself close up for the first time. This is most evident in controlled physical movement where the whole body must function co-ordinatively in motion.

It is natural when you first come to Taiji and Qi Gong that the new ideas and physical requirements seem insurmountable and quite alien, so it is really important at this stage to create a habit of attendance at class and to practise at home. Everyone has different problems and they do not get solved in class. They must be worked upon daily. As you build a vocabulary of movement you can also begin to deal with the problems. From the coarse and awkward gestures of the beginner a more fluid and refined skill, co-ordination and balance emerge, and comfort and physical relief develop as the physical and mental requirements become familiar and incorporated. Practice refines and distills the skills and the intelligence, as well as the gross and subtle energies, the cultivation of which is, after all, the real practice of Qi Gong.

The effects of Qi Gong are cumulative and constantly re-inform your practice, awareness and Qi Gong experience. It is as important to get it right at the beginning as it is through-out your Qi Gong journey, so never neglect the fundamental principles and methods of correct practice, whatever your level.

CHAPTER 13

So Where are You Now?

It is important to be able to place yourself within a long-term and developmental frame of Qi Gong and Taijiquan for it is easy to lose sight of both your own progress and where to place such disciplines in your life.

The first few years of study are often quite enthusiastic but when you feel you have reached a level of competence, it is not uncommon to wonder where you can go from there. There is no simple answer to this, beyond saying in a loud, clear voice, 'deeper'. Goal-oriented practice does not sit well with Qi Gong practice. In Taijiquan practised as a boxing art, for instance, it is much easier to judge progress objectively and determine where you are in your development. But with Qi Gong practice the sense of achievement and what that means can be much more elusive.

Diligent long-term practice and benefits often blend quietly into our ordinary life and our feelings and perception of ourselves. Indeed, they *should* become unself-consciously commonplace. This matches traditional practice. Like eating rice, your health maintenance is an everyday activity. Good practice should feel comfortable and familiar and somewhere you will always return to. It should not become a burden in life, nor should it be pursued in a dogged and overly ambitious way.

Nevertheless, the achievement of Qi Gong and Taijiquan are marked by at first distinctive, and later more subtle stages of development. You can only arrive at these if you are gently persistent in practice.

Everyone encounters problems at various stages and each person's problems may be different. Some of those problems will be easy to solve and others much more difficult, but no threshold can be crossed and no benefits gained unless the practice is done correctly with the right level of quiet and unassuming diligence.

Sadly, though, it is quite possible to practise Qi Gong and Taijiquan for a long time and still not 'catch' either the meaning or some of the profounder aspects that are at the heart of these arts. This is most often the result of a careless mental approach without real observation and internal investigation, or conversely of needing to achieve too much too quickly. Trying to run before you can walk is a common error. Such errors generally lead to frustration or a wrong perception of what is going on.

It is often also worth remembering that the pursuit of Qi Gong and Taijiquan is a major undertaking, and sometimes in your busy life you simply are not always able to give it the time and effort you would like. Going to the park every morning for two hours to practise with a master can be the case in China but is very different from two hours a week in a class. The other days may be taken up with your life and family commitments. When it becomes difficult you should take a break, and return when you have time and inclination. Trying to squeeze it in or not making enough time to do any practice is the same as not bothering to start.

It is also possible to flit like a butterfly among the many systems of Qi Gong and Chinese boxing, and among different teachers, picking up nuggets of information and forms from each. Sometimes, and for some people, this works, but you cannot keep it up without loss. In the end your mature practice must focus on what is achievable within your daily life, or you run the risk of not achieving proficiency or comfort with any of it.

The deeper the experience, the more it will encourage you to return to study. Critically, you must establish a practice as best you can within the constraints of your daily life. In addition you must direct your intelligence at that practice, for beyond the simple physical abilities and skills, that is the path to a fulfilling Qi Gong experience.

I have often found that it is when people are ill or in recovery and they have come to Qi Gong or Taijiquan specifically for their reputed benefits that practice is most appreciated and diligently kept up. It is when your condition requires such healing therapy that the benefits of practice are most evident. Its most overt rewards are muscular warmth and relaxation, as well as a quiet, comfortable feeling and a temporary relief from your daily concerns. Over a period of time this may turn into a feeling of increased Energy and a different quality of Energy. When focused they may feel both 'clear' and more 'vital' and this Energy can be applied to your daily tasks and can increase a sense of your physical self. The Qi Gong and Taiji community tells us that through practice youthful vigour can be retained longer, and can be recovered by older practitioners. It is the reward of practice.

In China it is not unusual to see octagenarians practising Qi Gong and Taijiquan in the early morning. Their vigour and stamina is beyond many younger practitioners who would be hard pressed to match some of their elders. It is wonderful to see such ability in older people, and I lament the fact that there is no such culture in the ageing population of the West. This must be considered an end in itself. Agility, flexibility, co-ordination, strength and, crucially, balance, are wonderful to see in the older generation, perhaps even more so than in the young. To be advanced in years and still to retain such capability are signs that the body and mind are well and healthy. It must be deeply satisfying at 80 to be able to twist and turn and move gracefully with balance and comfort. It is nothing short of inspirational. It is always worth reminding yourself of this, and if you need a goal, then this surely is the best one. It is good enough reason to learn and keep practising Qi Gong and Taijiquan. It gives us the chance to try to defy the inevitable degradation and decrepitude of old age.

Another of the great achievements of Qi Gong and Taijiquan is the sense of emotional well-being. This does not mean that your feathers can never be ruffled, but that you are more likely to maintain equanimity in the face of emotional difficulties and personal stress. Clarity devoid of excess emotional response is a quality that has really positive benefits in our daily lives, as we often meet with difficulties that can create both major and minor emotional disturbance. Having a practice that can balance or dissipate excess emotions and restore equanimity is truly beneficial. In fact it is a treasure and a secret weapon in the arsenal of modern survival. We no longer have to fight with swords on the battlefield as the Taiji masters of old may have done, but with our minds in the workplace, in our careers and interpersonal struggles and in the general hubbub and stress of modern life.

I have found that even in the face of the severest emotional upset like the death of a loved one, the mind and body can recover a sense of comfort and repose through practice. It not only offers relief from extreme emotions but can also alleviate the long-term residue of grief. Qi Gong and Taijiquan are methods of relief and release as well as rejuvenation.

In our modern world it seems hard to be totally autonomous or, for that matter, particularly individualistic any more, since we are all so 'linked up' and subject to the same influences. However, long practice of Qi Gong and Taiji does engender a sense of autonomy and individualistic independence. It is the ability to do something for yourself without plugging into a commercial network that is one of its charms in the modern world. Standing alone under a tree or practising in a quiet corner of a park does empower you in a way that few other activities do. It asserts your command of your personal condition and it gives you a window into what your condition is, as well as a way of rebalancing when needed. By just going to practise and by undertaking the discipline, you have already assumed a stance of self-help and self-cultivation. Training co-ordination, flexibility and especially balance, along with the discipline of focusing the mind and cultivating a quiescent mental landscape, at once connects you with your inner self. You forget ambitions, material needs and your daily problems.

This is not anaesthesia but a realisation of a bigger perspective, seeing yourself in a bigger world, an awesome and inspiring world governed by laws that were not made by man. It is a chance to resonate with nature and to dance to a deeper and profounder tune than that of our daily humdrum routine.

Qi Gong and Taiji engage us physically and mentally and often appear to be a puzzle of contradictory states. Solving those states is the way progress occurs, and dissolving the need to explain and re-siding in the experience alone is a lesson and a major contribution to the quality of our daily life. Regular practice fulfils both a deep sensual satisfaction in the mobility and co-ordination of our body and an intellectual satisfaction in the cultivation of the profound sense of integration and the palpable sense of heightened mental awareness reflected in the physical and the energetic. The movements of Qi Gong and Taiji at a mature level seem to access a deep and fulfilling emotional need in a way that feels like a distant memory being recovered and made real.

In the West self-cultivation is generally not linked to physical and mental well-being in the same way as in China, and it is certainly not linked to 'longevity' and the idea of retaining physical ability and mental faculties into old age. This has been handed over to the medical, pharmaceutical and cosmetic professions, though holistic therapies are gaining ground. Chinese traditional health culture is part of the daily life of many Chinese and is therefore more in the realm of personal responsibility and self-help. I expect that this may change with a new, more materially oriented generation, who will not have the time or the inclination to pursue the skills and knowledge that are the 'art of nourishing life and Eternal Spring', and which may not at first seem commensurate with the modern age. I believe, however, that those disciplines have as much or perhaps even greater value now than ever before.

Maturity in Qi Gong means a comfort and a natural and uncomplicated inclusion of practice in our daily life. There is no conflict about what is achieved and what is expected. In fact there is no need for expectations, since the deep lesson is to allow the benefits and lessons of Qi Gong to become apparent as and when they do, and in the end perhaps there is no lesson, but just residing in the state. This to me signals maturity in practice and learning.

All things appear simple and effortless in the hands of experts but it is important to remember that that apparently simple and effortless state results from long and serious effort. It is in the apparent simplicity and ordinariness of it all that its extraordinary value is concealed. This is when the knowledge and skill become an art.

Health, happiness and Eternal Spring

Regular and correct practice of Qi Gong and Taijiquan cultivates a new awareness of our 'wholeness' as well as our relationship with others, nature and the bigger forces that shape our lives and world. It is felt as a coherent energetic experience at the functional and physical and energetic levels as well as the emotional, intellectual and Spiritual levels.

The functional and physical characteristics of this experience are noticeable. There is a sense of increased co-ordination, mobility and balance. The whole body feels harmonious in stillness and movement. It is a natural feeling of comfort and ease. Consequently the body is more efficient, healthy, responsive, alert and sensitive. Qi Gong and Taijiquan restore a deep sense of pleasure and fulfilment in just being alive, breathing and moving. It is a natural, restorative and invigorating sensation.

The regular practice of Taijiquan and Qi Gong cultivates a quiescent mental state. The mindset is more accepting and open and less judgemental. It is simply aware and in-the-moment, and consequently less stressed by the jumble of thoughts and memories and all the little feelings and threads that constitute the habitual internal chatter that stretches into the past and projects into the future. That is our sense of self as a continuous entity. You come to realise that this sense of ourselves and our history is a burden that we carry with us unnecessarily. Through practice that burden dissolves. It loses its importance and although it remains our history, it no longer drags on us.

Taijiquan and Qi Gong generate emotional equanimity and consequently a clear mind. This can last as long as your daily practice or longer, or become a permanent mental climate. After practice there is a feeling of comfort, mild elation and deep relaxation. Long practice and keeping a Qi Gong awareness can become a more permanent state, clarity and comfort can be continuous. This becomes the backdrop aginst which all the subsequent dramas of your life are played out, but now you are more protected from the powerful and depleting effects of environmental and interpersonal events. It brings with it a mental lightness and a sense of personal and even Spiritual liberation.

Through practice, we also learn to be aware of ourselves on a much subtler energetic level where the sensation associated with the traditional concept of Qi becomes tangible. Sustained training in awareness and the accumulating and generating nature of the energetic self brings both a sense of robustness and energetic abundance, and free movement within the body. Practice generates healthy energetic distribution and internal balance. It is palpable. We are so used to an agitated and dispersed energetic state that we become attached to it as an aspect of who and what we are. The comfort of Taiji and Qi Gong is like calm after the storm. The currents are gentle and deep and healing, though it may take some time to accept and adjust to this new state.

To retain the Qi Gong state continuously is probably not possible for most of us, but even a gentle daily dip into the waters of Qi Gong and Taijiquan can thoroughly refresh all the parts and clear out the mental and physical cobwebs. It makes us happy and comfortable and rejuvenates, restores and invigorates.

In China, Qi Gong is renowned for its ability to impact favourably on all critical aspects of our physiology. It is used widely to 'cure' illness and promote healing and good health. It is alive and well on the streets and in the parks and in the hospitals. Its reputation rests on it positive healing and homeostatic effects. This reputation is as old as written history, and indeed undoubtedly older. The key health benefits identified by practitioners for centuries and more recently by modern researchers are considered to be the promotion of homeostasis and the functions of self-healing. This is brought about by an improvement in the immune system and heart function, a lowering of blood pressure, better circulation and efficient oxygenation, balanced blood chemistry, good lymphatic drainage, beneficial increase in endocrine function, more efficient cell metabolism, good digestion and waste elimination, and organ capacity, function and tone. This is an impressive list for something so apparently simple. Spiritual practice aside, the overall sense of increased vitality and well-being is what we can all expect from regular practice.

In China, Qi Gong and Taijiquan are practised to nourish life Energy (Yang Sheng) and for self-cultivation. Their aim is primarily to increase our potential for a healthy and happy life. The ultimate goal is Eternal Spring. This is not the longevity currently on offer by the medical profession or the pharmaceutical industry, where our years may be artificially extended but often at the expense of quality of life. In the West we all know that we are now more likely to live longer than at any other time in history, but at the same time, and here is the caveat, we are now more subject to lifestyle-related disease and cognitive deficiency and decrepitude in old age than ever before.

The practice of Qi Gong and Taijiquan allows us to participate in our own destiny and our own well-being and gives us the chance of a long and healthy life with dignity and a 'full pack of cards'. Not all of us can achieve this, and it is a sad fact that not many of us will bother to try. Sometimes there are just too many obstacles and demands on us for us to take the time to work on ourselves. Sometimes we come to this realisation too late. If we can accept responsibility for our own welfare and well-being from an early age, if we can have the opportunity and cultural encouragement to learn the arts of nourishing our life Energy and cultivating ourselves with Qi Gong and Taijiquan, we give ourselves a chance to stay healthy and happy for as long as possible. It is the chance of Eternal Spring.

CHAPTER 14

Experience Qi Gong – A Short Course for the Inquisitive

After all the words, it is perhaps this section, in the end, that is most valuable, since it is in the doing that benefits are accrued and knowledge is gained. This section is for the beginner and for those who perhaps have already dipped into the well and drawn some water but are still thirsty.

I have selected some very simple exercises that aim to offer you a taste of Qi Gong and which may also suffice as a daily regimen until you have found a teacher of merit and experience. I have kept my explanations simple and to the point.

The first methods concentrate on awareness of the physical state, structured relaxation and rooting. Next are simple gestures to develop qualities of movement and awareness of the directing mind. The next stage focuses on more dynamic integrated movement and balance. The vocabulary of movement and co-ordination is more demanding. Next there is the practice of Qi accumulation, Lower Dan Tian awareness and Qi circulation. This aims to generate and refine Jing (Essence) and Qi (Energy) and to build awareness of our energetic state. In addition it teaches a simple movement to propel and circulate Qi throughout the body and to smooth and harmonise blockage or uneven distribution. Finally we come to sitting. This is the last pinnacle to climb and is perhaps the highest and hardest. Its primary aim, at least in the beginning, is to refine the mental process (Shen) and to cultivate mental stillness. This is a long process, and so let it suffice at this stage to just undertake the practice and explore the inner state.

There are many ways to enter the house of Qi Gong and I should say that what and how I teach reflects the way of my master, Dr Li Li Qun. His paramount advice is always 'natural and comfortable'. So please take note if you begin practice.

The following methods are both simple and profound, but they are achievable by almost anyone who cares to try. You do not need to be a gymnast or a martial artist, and this is one of the great advantages of Qi Gong. It is open to young and old, the fit, the sick and the healing, or just anyone who wants to explore a new, healthy and possibly Spiritual practice. Remember that in Qi Gong the ordinary conceals the extraordinary and that the benefits accumulate through regular, correct and sincere practice. What you think you understand now will change with practice, and the longer you practise sincerely, the more you will understand and the deeper will be your knowledge. Not the knowledge of words, but the knowledge of experience. It can change the way you feel, see yourself and others and how you connect with and ride the waves of a lifetime.

Standing

Refer to the section 'Simply standing up' in Chapter 10 (pp.112–119) and become familiar with all the postural requirements for proper alignment.

Stand with your feet parallel and no wider apart than your shoulders (Fig. 1.1). Expand your arms outwards to the side slightly to create an open feeling in the armpit. Bend the elbows slightly to create a curve in the arms and point the hands downwards towards

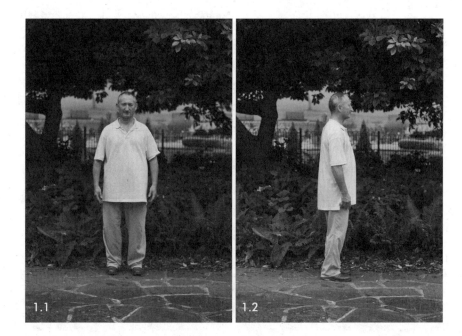

Exercise 1: Standing

the ground, and very, very slightly extend the fingers. Bend your knees slightly.

You must be relaxed and calm and feel comfortable and balanced. Your weight is spread evenly between the ball and heel of each foot, and equally between the feet. Imagine a plumb-line dropped from the sky passing through the top of your head (Bai Hui) and out between your legs (Hui Yin). This will align the Upper, Middle and Lower Dan Tian (Fig. 1.2). Feel your stability, feel your balance, and feel the downward sinking sensation of your muscles relaxing. At the same time feel the sensation of pushing against the ground and the upward rising resistance against the downward pull of gravity on your mass.

Allow your abdomen to relax; let go. As you inhale, your abdomen expands. Do not try to control your breath, but be aware of it. Observe yourself and feel the sense of yourself, now, in space, breathing, comfortable and perfectly balanced. Pay attention to the postural conditions of alignment and notice when and where tensions arise. Continually relax them. Key areas to notice are the shoulders, the lower back and the buttocks. Ensure that your knees are not pushed out forcefully.

Stand for at least five minutes and notice how your body tries to re-establish its habitual tensions. When you feel comfortable, become more aware of your breath and pay attention to the sensations of inhalation and exhalation. Close your eyes lightly (leave a small gap to let light in) and gently touch your tongue to the roof of your mouth behind your teeth. This connects the main energetic reservoirs of the back and the front (Yang and Yin). When your mind begins to wander, return your awareness to the sensations of your physical self, simply standing.

Building awareness

These exercises are included to give you a chance to practice simple upper body movement comprising lifting and lowering the arms and rotating the pelvis, shoulders and arms together. They are an opportunity to feel and refine how the directing mental intention (Yi Nian) converts to movement, and how movement awareness can in turn refine both the shape of the movement and the felt sensation of the movement.

First, assume the standing position, and when you are comfortable, decide to raise your arms up to shoulder height (Figs 2.1–2.3). You must aim to minimise muscle tension and not to raise your shoulders. Intention and movement will be simultaneous, but beware of habitual tensions and excessive use of local muscles. When your arms are at shoulder level, observe the tension in your chest, shoulders, lower back, buttocks and legs. Consciously relax them. The sense of relieving that tension is like a downward draining. The tension is not necessary or desirable. Notice how your body can support your extended arms, but in a more relaxed way. Lower your arms slowly and notice how the 'whole' body adjusts to the change.

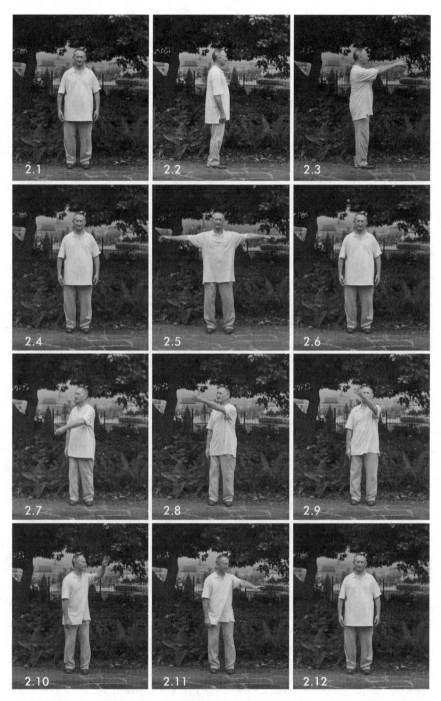

Exercise 2: Building awareness

In any movement your body must accommodate the change and re-assert its central balance (Zhong Ding). Repeat this movement and combine raising your arms with relaxed inhalation, and lowering arms with exhalation. Do not hold your breath but let movement follow the relaxed rhythm of your breathing. This practice brings a strong sense of energetic activity in the back. Return to the simple standing position. Do this exercise five to six times with relaxed breathing.

Initiate the thought to raise your arms to the side and to shoulder height. Relax your wrists and fingers (Fig 2.4). First rehearse the thought and the idea but do not move, then add the intention and gently, with the inhalation, raise your arms (Fig. 2.5). Relax your chest, back, shoulders, buttocks and legs. As with all Qi Gong movement, the external movement coincides with the rhythm of inhalation and exhalation. Do not stop or hold your breath. Lower your arms on exhalation but pay careful attention to how your body accommodates the change in movement and the distribution of tensions throughout the torso and legs. Compare this to the previous exercise. Let the movement feel light and comfortable. Return to the standing posture (Fig 2.6) and then do this movement five to six times with the breathing.

The next movement is a little more complicated and involves raising your left hand to the front right corner. Let the raised arm pull your shoulder as if stretching outward, and then let the shoulder pull the pelvis to turn simultaneously (Figs 2.7–2.8). Continue to raise your arm in a circular movement and bring it to the midline of the body (Fig. 2.9). The pelvis rotates with the shoulder to follow the hand. When the hand arrives at your centre line, the pelvis and shoulder have returned to face the front. Continue the hand movement in an arc to the left front corner, shoulders and pelvis following (Fig. 2.10). The hand prescibes a similar arc on the way down as it did on the way up, to return back to the front position (Figs 2.11–2.12). Use your line of sight to guide your hand as if movement follows your gaze. This movement should be done with both your right and left hand, five or six times each. Feel the co-ordinated hand, arm, shoulder and hip movement and the co-ordination of breath with the rising and falling of your hand and the rotation of your hips and shoulder.

Three co-ordinated movements to tonify, amplify and guide Qi flow

The following three exercises build upon relaxed and attentive awareness and guided movement. They use specific co-ordinated movements to harmonise, stimulate and amplify currents of Energy to move freely throughout the body and to emphasise energetic amplification to the arms and upper body. They also train a sense of 'rooting' and balance in motion, as well as opening up joints, lengthening muscles and 'unsticking' and activating connective tissue.

The first movement is the beginning form of the Taijiquan slow hand set. It mobilises up-and-down currents of Energy equally on both left and right sides of the body. It asserts our symmetry and balances both front and back.

The movement starts from the standing posture. The intention and will to move activates the action and guides the shape. Your hands rise in a circular and forward movement (Fig. 3.1) until they are just above shoulder height, and then follow an imaginary circle downwards (Figs 3.2–3.3). Rising and falling are co-ordinated with inhalation and exhalation and a gentle, smooth, fluid rhythm is accomplished through the increasingly relaxed posture and unforced co-ordination of breath and gesture.

The movement in Fig 3.4 harmonises upper (body and arms) with lower (legs) movement and develops co-ordination with the shifting of weight from one side to the other. First it must be done as a forward and backward single step from the standing position. When you are comfortable it can be done as a continuous forward walking exercise.

Start from the previous circular movement and as you begin the descending phase of the hands, stop them in front of your chest at heart height and rotate the palms inwards (Fig. 3.4). Take a moment to feel a connection between your hands and left and right sides, and the central body line. Relax your shoulders and on an exhalation turn the palms out and extend your left leg to step (Fig. 3.5). Make this step less than normal size so as to reduce muscular activity. Relax the extended leg and push forward with the back leg. Notice the gentle shift of weight as the previously 'empty' leg becomes weighted and 'solid'. Simultaneously extend your arms and hands. It should feel like pushing open a door but without any overtly obvious tension in your arms or legs (Fig. 3.6). When your arms are extended in this position, ensure that your shoulders are down and you are relaxed. Do not overextend. This stretched position is followed by turning over the palms, followed by a wide circular gesture that draws the hands apart (Fig. 3.7) and backwards to the shoulder line as the front and weighted leg simultaneously pushes your body back into a sitting-back posture (Fig. 3.8). The palms are naturally drawn into the chest by sinking your elbows, with your palms facing towards your chest. In the picture sequence I have re-peated this movement on one side (Figs 3.9–3.11). I recommend you try this on alternate sides, but always return to the standing posture (Fig. 3.12) before changing sides.

The fourth exercise is a variation of the well-known Cloud Hands movement that features strongly in the Taijiquan slow form. Actually it is very close to the Cloud Hands variation seen in the Wu Style fast form (Kuai Quan). It is a much more complicated movement than the previous two, since it requires a shift in weight combined with a waist rotation and a simultaneous rising and falling circular motion of the hands. Your hands do not have to be lifted as high as in the illustrations, and the rotations should be modest and aimed at achieving no more than a 90-degree rotation to the side from the front position. Your shoulders turn to follow the needs of the hand movement and circular extension, the pelvis follows and supports the turning of the shoulders. At first your shoulders and hips should

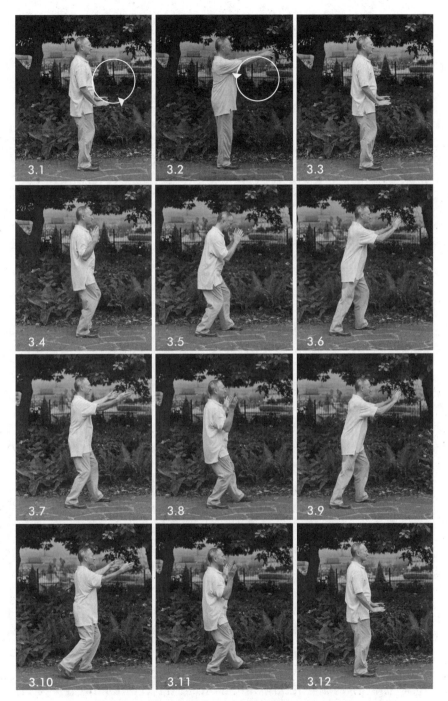

Exercise 3: Hand and Leg Coordination

rotate together. More advanced movement can accommodate a spi-ralling and twisting effect in the upper body, where shoulders rotate more than pelvis. This increases the squeezing and releasing effect in the torso. This frees 'stuck' muscle and connective tissue result-ing from energetic stagnation and stimulates the body's liquid envi-ronment. Additionally it massages and tonifies the five key internal organs – heart, lungs, liver, kidneys and spleen. There is a sense of Energy flooding the torso in waves and pushing through the arms, giving a sense of increased activity, first in one arm (lead hand) as it rises and reaches the apex of its arc and begins its descent, and then in the other hand and arm as it rises upwards. This is facilitated by the energetic pumping action of shifting weight. Freeing one side of weight allows increased mobility and relaxation in the hip, thus increasing the rotational ability of the pelvis. The continuous turning strengthens and activates the waist (Belt Channel) creating a powerful sense of upper and lower body integration.

Start from the the standing position and bring your hands, palms up, to the level of Lower Dan Tian (Fig. 4.1). Slowly raise them to Middle Dan Tian and then separate them, right side up and left down (Fig. 4.2). When your arms are comfortably extended (Fig. 4.3 – not too stretched, and do not lock the elbow joints) begin to rotate the waist and shift your weight into your left foot. Flex your right ankle slightly to raise your foot, keeping the heel on the ground (Fig. 4.4). Relax into the hip joint and then relax the big leg muscles. Your right hand describes a clockwise arc away from the body and to the side (Fig. 4.5) as you rotate. Do not push too far. Let your right hand begin to descend, and as it does so your left hand begins to rise up, led by the fingers to describe an anti-clockwise arc. Rotate your waist and shoulders to follow your left hand back to the centre line of the body (Fig. 4.6). Bring your weight back to an even distribution between both feet (Fig. 4.7). Continue to rotate and follow the left hand to the left side. Shift weight into your right foot and free your left hip (Fig. 4.8). As the left hand descends, the right hand rises and returns in an arc to the centre (Figs 4.9–4.11) and then to the starting position by allowing the upper hand to drop slightly down the body centre line to the level of the lower hand (Fig 4.12). Both hands then turn up and rise slightly, then turn over and press down, separate and fall to the sides. Repeat this five or six times with natural and easy breaths. Inhalation follows the rising of the left hand and exhalation the descent of that hand. Be relaxed and comfortable.

The fifth exercise is the Qi accumulation, circulation and closing form. This form is a still, meditational standing posture that is a fundamental Qi Gong posture. It is primarily used to focus mental activity on Lower Dan Tian, to regulate abdominal breathing and to enter a state of deep relaxation. This posture is used to cultivate and energise the lower energetic centre and to facilitate the conservation and transformation of 'Pre-Heavenly' Essence (Jing) and Energy (Qi). It is simple and profound.

Simply take up the posture and follow all the postural instruction. Cover Lower Dan Tian with both hands (Fig. 5.1) so as to bring a sense of comfort and warmth in the Lower Dan Tian. Focus your attention on this field and pay attention to your breathing and the rise and fall of your abdomen. Feel comfortable and relaxed. You can hold this posture for five or more minutes while you feel the changing sensations and adjustments of your body entering a state of relaxation. It can help to count your exhalations until your mental activity has become focused. Like all Qi Gong, the benefits of this practice are acquired over a period of time, so do not expect mind-blowing revelations. Assume the practice and allow the body to achieve a natural feeling of balance and an internal climate of comfort. Allow the early coarse sensations to reveal subtle changes and feelings.

This movement follows on from the standing posture and requires you to bring your attention from the Lower Dan Tian to Yong Quan in the base of your feet, located in line with the second toe and just behind the ball of the foot, in the hollow created when the toes are curled up and the foot flexed. Exhale and drop your hands to the side (Fig. 5.2), inhale and begin to lift them in a circle (Fig. 5.3). Shift your attention to the point Lao Gong in the centre of the

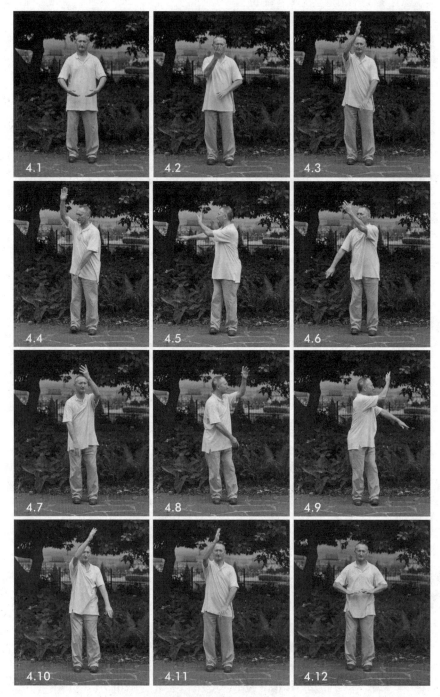

Exercise 4: Cloud Hands

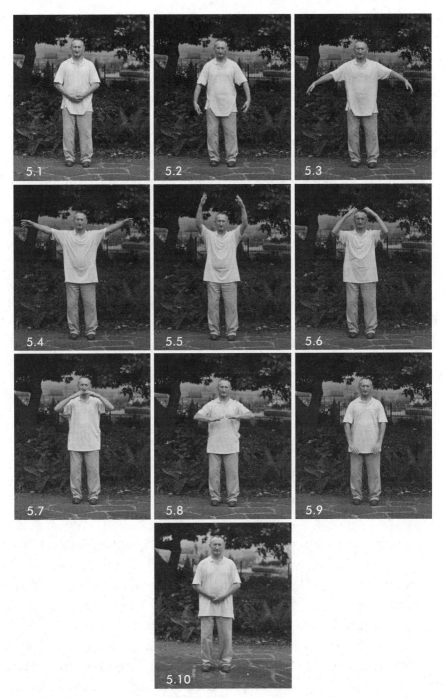

Exercise 5: Qi accumulation, circulation and closing form

palms of your hands. When the arms are shoulder height or slightly above (keep your shoulder joints open and relaxed), fold from the elbows (Fig. 5.5) and point the palms at the crown of your head (Bai Hui) (Fig. 5.6). Exhale and bring your arms down the front line of the body with palms facing down (Figs 5.7–5.8). Mentally follow the path of the hands down to Lower Dan Tian (Fig. 5.9) and simultaneously draw a path from Bai Hui down the front line of the body with your awareness. Continue that path down to the soles of your feet to complete the exhalation. Follow the breath, do not force anything and do not hold your breath. After the first exercise your breath will be calmed. It is important to maintain that state and follow it gently. Excessive attention will scatter your Energy. Be calm and feel comfortable and at ease. There is no pressure to achieve or win and no one to impress.

This circulation can be done five to ten or more times, but it is important not to stress the shoulder muscles. This exercise stimulates what is known as the Large Heavenly Circuit and smooths the upward and downward flow of Energy. It harmonises movement and breath and calms the mental activity.

On completion of this set of Qi Gong it is important to assume the closing posture (Fig. 5.10). Re-focus your mind on Dan Tian and ensure a fully relaxed and properly structured posture.

Sitting meditation

Be sure to read the section on meditation in Chapter 10 (pp. 133–139) before you begin this practice. Aim at 20–25 minutes sitting if possible, but do not torture yourself. Try to make a commitment to 100 days of practice. This will give you the best chance of success. Find a quiet place and make it your regular spot.

Sit comfortably so that there is no stress or tension in your legs. Touch your tongue to the roof of your mouth, assert the Bai Hui to Hui Yin plumb-line and relax your shoulders and abdomen. Breathe naturally and comfortably, allowing your abdomen to expand on

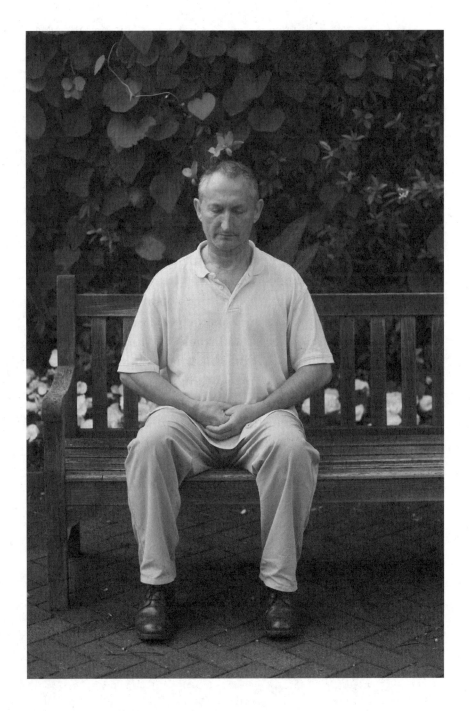

Exercise 6: Sitting meditation

inhalation and naturally deflate on exhalation. Fold your hands together and lower your eyelids.

Begin by counting the exhalations. This will focus your attention and quieten excessive mental activity, inner dialogue and the distraction of external sounds and local activity. Try at least 50 counts. Your breaths will become naturally soft, quiet, long, deep and equal in length, but do not force this. If your attention wanders, then bring it back to the counting.

At the end of the 50 breaths feel the rhythm of your inhalation and exhalation and then, for another 50 counts, on the inhalation feel as if oxygen (Qi) is permeating every cell of your body. On the exhalation feel as if all stale and stagnant Energy leaves you. It is like opening the windows in a stuffy house. Feel cleansed and refreshed. After a while you may find that you naturally forget what you are doing and slip into a deep and quiet state. Just reside in this experience and rest in the peace and comfort of the moment.

You will emerge naturally from this when you become aware of yourself and what you are doing and thinking. The more you practise, the deeper and the longer this experience will last. Eventually you may feel that a deep quietness becomes part of your daily life.

None of this happens overnight, but remember each meditation is a step on a journey of self-cultivation. Let each step unfold without fixed expectations or rigid goals. Be natural and unself-conscious about it, but make a commitment to stick at it.

References

Fung, Y.L. (1997) translation of Chuang Tzu's *A Taoist Classic*. Beijing: Foreign Languages Press.

Herrigel, E. (1989) *Zen in the Art of Archery*. New York: Vintage Books.

Lau, D.C. (1963) translation of Lao Tzu's *Tao Te Ching*. London: Penguin Group.

Ma, Y.L. Zee, W. (1990). *Wu Style Tai Chi Chuan Push Hands*. Hong Kong: Shanghai Book Co. Ltd.

Ni, M.S. (1995) *The Yellow Emperor's Classic of Medicine*. Boston/London: Shambala.

Suzuki, D.T. (1961) *Essays in Zen Buddhism*. New York: Grove.

Suzuki, D.T. (1964) An Introduction to Zen Buddhism. New York: Grove Press.

Wang X. and Moffett. J.P. (1994) *Traditional Chinese Therapeutic Exercises – Standing Pole*. Beijing: Foreign Language Press.

Watts, A. (1997) *Tao – The Watercourse Way with Al Chung-Liang* Hua. New York: Pantheon.

Watts, A. (1999) *The Way of Zen* (Vintage Spiritual Classic). New York: Vintage Books.

Wilhelm, R. (trans.) (1965) *The I Ching or Book of Changes* (third edn). London: Routledge and Kegan Paul.

Index